DIABETES MANAGEMENT

Step by Step

Michael H. Drucquer
DCH, DRCOG, MRCGP
General Practitioner
South Wigston Health Centre
Leicester, UK

Paul G. McNally
MD, FRCP
Consultant Physician
Leicester Royal Infirmary
Leicester, UK

b

**Blackwell
Science**

First published 1998
Reprinted 1999

Set by Excel Typesetters Co., Hong Kong
Printed and bound in Great Britain
at the Alden Press, Oxford and Northampton

DISTRIBUTORS

Marston Book Services Ltd
PO Box 269
Abingdon, Oxon OX14 4YN
(*Orders*: Tel: 01235 465500
        Fax: 01235 465555)

USA
Blackwell Science, Inc.
Commerce Place
350 Main Street
Malden, MA 02148 5018
(*Orders*: Tel: 800 759 6102
        781 388 8250
    Fax: 781 388 8255)

Canada
Login Brothers Book Company
324 Saulteaux Crescent
Winnipeg, Manitoba, R3J 3T2
(*Orders*: Tel: 204 837-2987)

Australia
Blackwell Science Pty Ltd
54 University Street
Carlton, Victoria 3053
(*Orders*: Tel: 3 9347 0300
        Fax: 3 9347 5001)

A catalogue record for this title
is available from the British Library
and the Library of Congress

ISBN 0-632-048484

For further information on
Blackwell Science, visit our website:
www.blackwell-science.com

The Blackwell Science logo is a
trade mark of Blackwell Science Ltd,
registered at the United Kingdom
Trade Marks Registry

DIABETES
MANAGEMENT
Step by Step

Contents

Self-Assessment Questionnaire

Appendices

Colour plates fall between pp. 22 and 23

Preface

This workbook is designed for health care professionals who are working or are about to work with patients who have diabetes and feel that they may have gaps in their knowledge and expertise.

The idea for it came when one of us (M.H.D.) had planned a tutorial with a trainee general practitioner with the aim of 'doing diabetes'. Although we had textbooks, articles, guidelines and formularies to work with we found it difficult to know where to start and consequently struggled to get to grips with the subject. What we felt was needed was a practical learning guide for diabetes which would take us through the subject in a logical sequence but which, by setting tasks and posing questions, would avoid spoon-feeding and overload of information.

Foremost in our minds is the realisation that the patients we see in our clinics and surgeries most frequently present a mixture of physical, psychological and social problems which makes the implementation of ideal management guidelines a difficult task. Therefore, we have tried to make the factual component of the workbook as unambiguous and straightforward as possible, whilst addressing some of the complexities of the modern management of diabetes through real life clinical scenarios.

We all find the subject of diabetes a daunting one. There are many clinical situations, such as the newly diagnosed diabetic patient or the ill insulin dependent patient, which health care professionals might understandably approach with less than complete confidence. We hope this book makes your task an easier one.

Acknowledgements
We thank: The Department of Community Medicine, Monash University, Melbourne, for providing M.H.D. with the facilities for researching this book whilst on sabbatical there; Professor John Murtagh, Head of Department, for his help and encouragement; Jenny Green for word processing the first draft from barely legible handwritten copy; Jane Sapsford for her patience in word processing the many amendments and additions and Dr Peter Swift for his help in drafting the 'Diabetes in children' section.

Michael H Drucquer
Paul G McNally

Abbreviations

ACE	Angiotensin converting enzyme
BDA	British Diabetic Association
BG	Blood glucose
BMI	Body mass index
DCCT	The Diabetes Control and Complications Trial
GFR	Glomerular filtration rate
HbA1(c)	Haemoglobin A1(c) (glycosylated)
HDL	High density lipoprotein
IDDM	Insulin dependent diabetes mellitus
IHD	Ischaemic heart disease
LDL	Low density lipoprotein
NIDDM	Non-insulin dependent diabetes mellitus
OHA	Oral hypoglycaemic agent
SBGM	Self blood glucose monitoring
U & Es	Urea and electrolytes

How to use this workbook

The workbook is divided into three sections: 25 skill topics, 13 clinical scenarios and a self-assessment questionnaire.

- *Skill topics*. These are concise clinical guidance sheets aimed at facilitating basic day to day management. You may choose to read them selectively as it is intended that the next two sections will encourage you to refer back to them for key points. See contents list page v.
- *Clinical scenarios*. These real life clinical situations are intended to be thought provoking and to address some of the grey areas of patient management. You can do them on your own but they have worked well as a stimulus for group discussion or as a starting point for trainer/trainee tutorials.
- *Self-assessment questionnaire*. You may wish to do the questionnaire blind to gauge the level of your expertise but more importantly we see it as a learning exercise to complement the scenarios; for this reason the answers come with expanded explanations. Once again, it is intended that you will be encouraged to refer back to the skill topics for further information.

There are therefore three main ways in which you may wish to use the workbook.

Method 1. Read through the skill topics in greater or lesser detail, but concentrate on the scenarios and questionnaire with frequent revisiting of skill topics.

Method 2. If you are short of time, refer to the 'quick learning planner' on page 103 and pick out those questions you might find challenging. Go straight to the section of the workbook indicated.

Method 3. Patient based. You may prefer an initial read of the skill topics and then to refer to them as problem patients arise in your clinical practice. We believe however, that most benefit will be gained from the workbook by tackling all or some of the scenarios and questionnaire.

DIABETES
SKILL TOPICS

How to diagnose diabetes

The diagnosis of diabetes is straightforward in most cases as patients usually present with the following classic symptoms and a raised blood glucose in the diagnostic range (Tables 1.1 & 1.2).

- Polyuria.
- Polydipsia.
- Weight loss.

However, patients may present with other symptoms or signs and a diagnosis of diabetes should be considered when the following occur:

- recurrent skin infections, balanitis, pruritis vulvae, thrush;
- urinary incontinence, nocturia, bedwetting in children;
- peripheral vascular disease, foot ulceration;
- IHD and cerebrovascular events;
- peripheral neuropathy, erectile dysfunction;
- lethargy.

Diagnostic criteria

- In a symptomatic patient, diabetes is diagnosed by demonstrating a single raised value in the diagnostic range (see below) using either a random blood glucose or a fasting blood glucose. In the absence of symptoms at least two blood glucose readings in the diagnostic range should be documented.
- The number of formal glucose tolerance tests can be reduced by taking random samples about 2 hours after a main meal. As fasting blood glucose levels may be within the normal range at diagnosis, a random sample may provide more information.
- Remember that the diagnostic criteria vary depending on whether the blood sample is whole blood or plasma (whole blood glucose values are 10–15% lower than plasma levels) and whether it is venous or capillary (capillary glucose levels are about 10% higher than venous). Venous blood samples are usually taken and the results shown below are venous plasma glucose levels.
- 1998 is likely to see two important changes to the diagnostic criteria with the aim of enabling the earlier detection of diabetic complications. Firstly, the introduction of a new category of abnormality for fasting levels between 6.1 and 6.9 mmol/l termed 'impaired fasting glucose' and

Table 1.1 Interpretation of glucose values using venous plasma glucose.

		Venous plasma glucose (mmol/l)	Interpretation
Normal values	Fasting Random	<6.1 and <7.0	Normal values. Diabetes most unlikely
Diabetes	Fasting Random	>7.0 or 11.1	Diabetes confirmed No glucose tolerance test required
Diagnosis uncertain	Random	7.0 to <11.1	Fasting glucose required or glucose tolerance test
Impaired glucose tolerance	Fasting	6.1–6.9	Impaired fasting glucose

Table 1.2 Diagnostic criteria following a standard glucose tolerance test. (New criteria 1998.)

		Venous plasma glucose (mmol/l)	Interpretation
Normal values	Fasting 2 hour	<6.1 and <7.8	Normal values
Diabetes	Fasting 2 hour	>7.0 or <11.1	Diabetes confirmed
Impaired glucose tolerance	Fasting	6.1–6.9	Impaired fasting glucose
Impaired glucose tolerance	2 hour	>7.8 to <11.1	Impaired glucose tolerance

secondly a lowering of the threshold for diagnosis of diabetes on fasting samples from 7.8 to 7.0 mmol/l.

• Patients with borderline results should undergo a glucose tolerance test. This test can be simplified by measuring only a fasting and 2 hour blood glucose level. The patient should maintain a normal unrestricted diet prior to the test and should fast for at least 10 hours overnight (water is allowed). Smoking and strenuous activities during the test are not permitted. The glucose load may be given as glucose 75 g mixed with 250–300 ml of water or alternatively as 400 ml of a glucose based drink.

• Samples should be measured using a laboratory method and *not* using test strips.

• Impaired glucose tolerance *is* important. Up to 10–25% will progress to diabetes over the next 5 years. Those with continuing impaired glucose tolerance have a higher prevalence of IHD, peripheral vascular disease and strokes. Patients are advised on lifestyle changes and a small proportion return to normal glucose tolerance. The glucose tolerance test should be repeated annually and the patient advised to see his or her general practitioner if symptoms develop.

Key points
- Diabetes cannot be diagnosed by simply detecting glycosuria.
- Very few patients require a glucose tolerance test!
- Do not diagnose diabetes using a glycosylated haemoglobin.
- Know which glucose your local laboratory reports.

See also:
Questionnaire, page 79, Diagnosis.

Initial management step by step

Having diagnosed diabetes you must now decide what sort of diabetes the patient has and how you are going to treat it.

For those of you who hate flow charts (see next page) here is a simple sequence to follow when confronted with a newly diagnosed patient.

For the management of newly diagnosed children see Skill Topic 22.

• Admit patient to hospital if severely symptomatic or ill with vomiting, dehydration, drowsiness or disordered (acidotic) breathing.

• If hospital admission not indicated but *clinical picture suggests IDDM* discuss same day with diabetologist with a view to outpatient initiation of insulin. Moderate or severe ketonuria *or* weight loss are highly suggestive of IDDM (see Scenario 1).

• *If clinical picture suggests NIDDM* pursue a 12 week trial of diet (see Scenario 2). Monitor patient carefully during this phase (weekly for 2 weeks then monthly) checking for urinary ketones or excessive weight loss. Reconsider need for insulin if clinical state deteriorates.

• It may be necessary to abandon the 12 week dietary trial and start an oral hypoglycaemic agent early, if the patient remains symptomatic or if the fasting blood glucose remains persistently high (>15 mmol/l). However, symptoms can take several weeks to settle particularly if the patient is obese.

• If fasting venous blood glucose is >7 mmol/l or glycosylated haemoglobin (HbA1 or HbA1c) above normal range after the 12 week dietary trial, start an OHA (see Skill Topic 6, Starting oral hypoglycaemic agents). A higher threshold is acceptable in the elderly in whom reasonable control may be taken as a fasting glucose of 7–9 mmol/l.

See also:

Scenarios 1 & 2
Questionnaire, page 80, Initial management.

Initial management flow chart

Points

1 Monitor the patient carefully in the initial dietary phase for the development of ketonuria or excessive weight loss. If these occur reconsider the need for insulin.

2 Fasting venous plasma glucose of <7 mmol/l after 12 weeks of diet indicates good control. A higher level would be acceptable in the elderly.

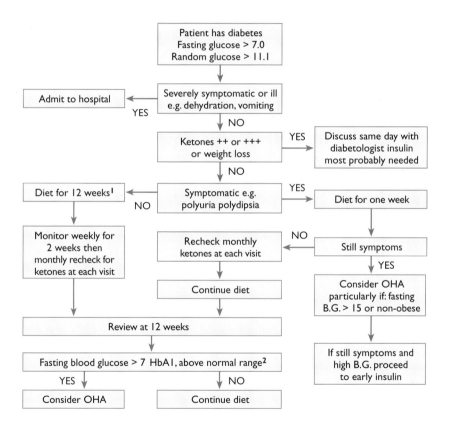

Diet

The recommended diabetic diet has undergone considerable changes in the past 15 years. The exchange system, based on weighed carbohydrate portions has been superseded by a much more user friendly, flexible and less restrictive diet which is very similar to the ideal recommended for the whole population.

The three main aims of the diabetic diet are:

1 to improve glycaemic control and prevent microvascular complications;

2 to improve the cardiovascular risk factors profile;

3 to avoid hypoglycaemia.

These aims can be achieved by following some simple guidelines in the following areas.

• *Weight control.* Lowering the BMI of obese patients to within the normal range will decrease insulin resistance and improve their lipid profile. Even small weight reductions are worthwhile.

• *Starchy carbohydrate.* The current recommendations are that 50% of calories should derive from carbohydrate, 30–35% from fat and 10–15% from protein. In practice these bare figures necessitate that every meal should be starch based with larger than accustomed quantities of potato, pasta, rice, bread and chapatis. Preferably, the starch should be in 'slow release' form from sources high in natural fibre such as wholemeal products and from food high in soluble fibre such as beans, pulses, fruits and oats.

• *Fat.* Total fat intake should be reduced using small quantities of monounsaturated fats, e.g. olive oil or polyunsaturated fats wherever possible. Lean meats can be eaten even as part of a calorie controlled diet.

• *Sugar.* A total ban on sugar is impractical and unnecessary. Sugar which occurs naturally in foods like fresh fruit and that added to bought savoury foods such as tomato ketchup or baked beans is not generally enough to upset control, particularly if low sugar varieties are chosen. Non-obese patients can allow themselves up to 25 g of additional sucrose per day, as might be found in biscuits, cakes or sugary spreads, best taken along with other high fibre food, and providing that the extra 100 kcal that this will provide is taken into account in the day's total calorie intake.

• *Sweeteners.* Sorbitol and fructose are not suitable as they are highly calorific and are laxative in large amounts. Saccharin and aspartame are useful sweeteners but are neutralised by cooking.

• So called '*diabetic foods*'. These should be *avoided*. Although low in sucrose, they are high in total calories and are expensive.

• *Snacks*. Insulin treated patients need three medium sized meals per day plus snacks at mid morning, mid afternoon and before bed. This is essential to smooth control and avoid 'hypos'. Suitable snacks are fruit, plain biscuits, wholemeal toast, muesli bars or low fat crisps.

• *Alcohol*. Diabetic patients are advised to consume no more than 21 units per week for men and 14 units for women but these levels should be halved if there is poor control or obesity. Alcohol not only increases the risk of hypoglycaemia, which can be delayed, but also impairs the body's ability to release glucose from the liver in the event of it occurring. It is best for patients to stick to dry wines and low alcohol beers and to consume them with a meal.

In practice

• All newly diagnosed patients with diabetes should be seen by a dietician. Until seen, use a brief guidance diet sheet provided by your dietician or obtained from the BDA who do a useful tear off pad.

• If appropriate, set a realistic weight reduction target of not more than 1–2 kg per month. (Depends on age and activity level.)

• Tell patients what to do about sugar intake (see above). They will expect some guidance on this from the start and will worry enormously if you do not give it.

See also:

Questionnaire, page 80, Diet.

Oral hypoglycaemic agents

Oral hypoglycaemic agents should be introduced only after a reasonable dietary trial and not at diagnosis (see Skill Topic 2, Initial management step by step).

There are three main classes.

1 Biguanides.
2 Sulphonylureas.
3 Alpha glucosidase inhibitors.

Biguanides

- Metformin is the only biguanide in use.
- Works by reducing hepatic glucose output, by enhancing peripheral glucose uptake by muscle and by reducing appetite.
- Is the drug of choice for obese patients.
- Its gastrointestinal side-effects (diarrhoea, flatulence and nausea) may be limited by starting at a low dose (500 mg daily) and by giving with food.
- Should be avoided in patients with renal impairment, in cardiac or liver failure, in patients with alcohol abuse and in acute myocardial infarction as there is a risk of lactic acidosis.

Sulphonylureas

- Agents in use include tolbutamide, glipizide, gliclazide and glibenclamide.
- Work by stimulating pancreatic beta-cells to release insulin.
- Are the drug of choice in normal or underweight patients and should be gradually increased from a low starting dose.
- The most serious side-effect is hypoglycaemia to which the elderly and patients with renal impairment are prone, particularly if drugs with a long half life or which are renally excreted are prescribed such as glibenclamide or chlorpropamide.
- Tolbutamide and gliclazide are metabolised by the liver and are less likely to cause hypoglycaemia.
- Weight gain is often an unwanted side-effect.
- Can be given in combination with metformin.

Alpha glucosidase inhibitors (acarbose)

• Works by delaying absorption of glucose from carbohydrate containing foods.

• Main side-effects are flatulence and diarrhoea.

• Start with a low dose to minimise symptoms (50 mg once daily) and give with food.

• Can be used in conjunction with both metformin and sulphonylureas.

See also:

Questionnaire, page 81, Oral hypoglycaemic agents.

Starting oral hypoglycaemic agents

1 Body mass index is calculated by dividing the weight in kilograms by the square of the height in metres.

2 Avoid long-acting sulphonylureas such as glibenclamide and chlorpropramide particularly in the elderly.

3 Acarbose is a useful alternative if intolerant of metformin. It can also be used as triple therapy in combination with metformin and a sulphonylurea.

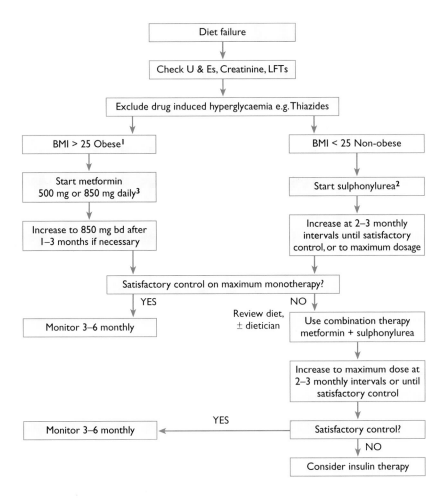

Insulin therapy

Which insulin?
- New patients are most usually started on genetically engineered human insulins which have low antigenicity and cause less lipoatrophy. Highly purified animal insulins remain available for patients who have been stable on them for many years.
- Soluble or clear insulins are short acting; cloudy isophane insulins are intermediate acting. Premixed preparations (soluble 30%, isophane 70%) aid convenience but are less flexible if patient requires more or less soluble or isophane. Lispro is a new soluble insulin analogue with a shorter duration and faster onset of action which theoretically gives improved postprandial control. It can be injected immediately before eating and may cause less hypoglycaemia.

How much insulin?
- The usual total dose of insulin is between 0.5 and 1 unit/kg/day although it is usual to work up slowly from a starting dose of 0.25 unit/kg/day.
- When stabilised, most patients require about 60% of total insulin in the morning and 40% in the evening. However, the insulin dosing regimen needs to be individually tailored—many patients take 50% morning and evening.
- Overweight patients often need more insulin due to insulin resistance. Combination therapy with metformin may limit weight gain and reduce the amount of insulin required by decreasing insulin resistance.

What is the advised injection technique?
- Injections are given subcutaneously into pinched-up skin. Suitable areas are abdomen, anterior thighs, buttocks and arms. It is best to stick to one area but to rotate the site of injections within it from day to day.
- Injections are best given 15–20 minutes before a meal.

Insulin for IDDM patients
There are two main regimens.
1 A twice daily mixture of a short-acting (clear soluble) and intermediate-acting (cloudy isophane) insulin.

2 The basal bolus regimen. Particularly suitable for patients with irregular meal times or hectic lifestyles this regimen consists of an intermediate-acting insulin at bed time with soluble, short-acting insulin before each main meal. Disposable pen injections avoid the need to carry around separate vials and syringes and are quicker to use but the basic injection technique remains the same. A useful feature of pen injectors is that they can be fitted with the very fine 30G needle.

Self monitoring of blood glucose with or without a meter is recommended for IDDM patients at least once daily. Testing times should be varied with the majority preprandial or at bed time. See Skill Topic 8, Targets for control, and page 82 of the Self-assessment questionnaire for more information on monitoring and dosage adjustment.

Insulin for NIDDM patients

At least 35% of NIDDM patients eventually require insulin. The average general practice of 2000 patients will have to transfer about two NIDDM patients to insulin each year.

The *indications* for starting insulin in a NIDDM patient are:

• Persistent hyperglycaemia and inadequate control despite maximal oral therapy. Strict targets do not apply to elderly or infirm patients or to those with hypoglycaemic unawareness. (See Skill Topic 8 and Scenario 7.)

• Weight loss due to hyperglycaemia or ketosis.

• Intercurrent illness. (Temporary indication usually undertaken in hospital.)

• Persistent diabetes related symptoms or complications despite maximal oral therapy. Some patients who have vague symptoms of ill health including lethargy and muscle weakness with only moderate hyperglycaemia can respond well to insulin, perhaps initially on a trial basis. Up to 70% of patients report an increase in well-being after transferring to insulin.

Key points
- Insulin is not a substitute for lifestyle modification. Giving insulin to obese patients usually makes them more obese. Satisfactory control can then be difficult to achieve. However, if biochemical control is still not achieved after dietary review and patient education, insulin should be advised. Metformin or acarbose can be given in combination with insulin in obese patients. (See Skill Topic 5, Oral hypoglycaemic agents.)
- Before transferring a non-insulin dependent patient to insulin think of other causes of poor control such as dietary non-compliance, occult infection or thyroid problems.

Which regimen for NIDDM patients?

• Intermediate-acting isophane insulin can work well on its own in NIDDM patients but a soluble component is often needed. If an isophane is used on its own the mid-morning and mid-afternoon snacks which are necessary in patients on rapid-acting soluble insulin, can be reduced and the timing of meals is less critical, although the pre-bedtime snack remains obligatory.

• Soluble insulin can be added if postprandial hyperglycaemia 2 hours after a meal is excessive (>10 mmol/l).

• A few elderly patients can be managed on once daily lente insulin. Lente insulins are complexed with zinc to form a long-acting suspension and cannot be mixed with soluble insulin.

In practice: most general practitioners refer NIDDM patients to the specialist Diabetes Team for initiation of insulin therapy. Transferring back to general practitioner care once therapy is established is nearly always possible. However, if you prefer to do it yourself, or the patient is unhappy to go to hospital, here is a simple system:

• Insulin, syringes, needle clipper, blood testing lancets and strips are pre-scribed. Patient is advised about availability of finger-prick devices which make capillary blood sampling more comfortable. However, patients may continue urine testing if they do not wish to change.

• Patient does not take any oral hypoglycaemic agents on day of starting insulin.

• Patient attends surgery at 8.30 a.m. bringing breakfast.

• Patient is shown how to give insulin injection, then has breakfast.

• Work through the patient education checklist (see Scenario 3) backed up by suitable written material.

• Review patient at 5.30 p.m., measure blood glucose and give second insulin.

• Injections are supervised by practice nurse until it is clear that technique is satisfactory.

• Patient attends at least every other day for first week and then at least weekly for 4 weeks to assess control and answer questions.

• Start low, go slow. There is no rush to achieve adequate control—this may take several weeks. Start with 8–10 units twice daily. Increase by 2–4 units every 2–3 days according to capillary blood glucose values or urinalysis.

See also:
   Scenarios 3, 4, 5 & 7
   Questionnaire pages 81–83.

Targets for control

Blood glucose targets vary slightly from country to country and often from year to year! The aim of therapy is to achieve the best possible gly-caemic control without compromising quality of life or causing adverse side-effects. Effective therapy for co-existent vascular risk factors should also form part of the overall management plan.

Note that:
• The presence of complications (micro or macro) lowers the threshold for intervention.
• The American Diabetes Association now recommends a bedtime blood glucose of up to 7.8 mmol/l. This slight relaxation of control is in view of the DCCT (see Appendix 1) during which strict goals were associated with a 3-fold increase in hypoglycaemia.
• Strict targets need not apply to the elderly, infirm patients or patients with hypoglycaemic unawareness.
• It is essential to check reference values of HbA1 and HbA1c from your local laboratory as they vary according to the technique used. Many laboratories are now switching from HbA1 to HbA1c.

	Normal	Acceptable	High risk
Fasting and preprandial (mmol/l)	4–7	<8	>8
2 hours postprandial (mmol/l)	<8	8–10	>10
HbAl (per cent)	4–8.5	≤9.5	>9.5
HbAlc (per cent)	3–6.5	≤7.5	>7.5
Glycosuria	Negative	≤0.5%	>0.5%
Total cholesterol	<5.2 mmol/l	≤6.5 mmol/l	>6.5 mmol/l
LDL-cholesterol	<3.4 mmol/l	≤4.1 mmol/l	>4.1 mmol/l
HDL-cholesterol	1.1 mmol/l	≥0.9 mmol/l	<0.9 mmol/l
Fasting triglycerides	<1.7 mmol/l	≤2.2 mmol/l	>2.2 mmol/l
Body mass index	Male 20–25	<27	>27
	Female 19–24	<26	>26

(Adapted from *Recommendations for the Management of Diabetes in Primary Care* published by the BDA, 1997)

- If assessing control in NIDDM using fasting venous plasma, targets are as for preprandial levels above.
- Encourage patients to stop smoking and take exercise.
- Discussion and negotiation of targets with patients are always preferable to inappropriate one-sided lectures—not all patients are able or willing to achieve the ideal.

Retinopathy

It is hard to learn the theory and practice of screening for diabetic retinopathy from textbooks. There are conflicting classifications and an over-reliance on poorly explained pathological terms. However, any general practitioner caring for diabetic patients will need to do at least some fundal examination and the following is an attempt to simplify the procedures. There is no substitute, however, for learning from real patients and the reader is advised if possible to attend a hospital retinal clinic or one of the practical courses available several times a year at different centres. (The BDA keep an up to date list of courses which is sent out regularly to members of their professional section.)

Diabetic retinopathy
- Is the commonest cause of blindness in those age <65 years in the UK.
- Causes blindness in 2% of diabetics.
- Is caused by retinal ischaemia and oedema.
- Is largely treatable by laser photocoagulation.
- Is best treated before visual loss occurs.

Diabetic retinopathy may be classified into four broad groups.
1 Background retinopathy.
2 Maculopathy.
3 Preproliferative retinopathy. } Require hospital referral.
4 Proliferative retinopathy.

Key point
Remember that visual loss can be caused by cataract as well as retinopathy.

Background retinopathy (Plate 1, facing page 22)
Features include
- Microaneurysms.
- Small 'blot' haemorrhages.

• Hard exudates. These have a bright, 'slapped-on' appearance with a distinct edge. Sometimes described as waxy. Light yellow in colour. Caused by capillary leakage of lipoproteins.

Maculopathy (Plate 2, facing page 22)
The commonest cause of diabetic blindness; it results in a gradual misting of vision with a sparing of peripheral vision. It is particularly common in NIDDM. It is best to think of it as background retinopathy occurring within one disc diameter of the macula.
Features include:
• exudates and/or haemorrhages at or around the macula;
• exudates often in a ring around and close to the macula, so-called circinate exudates;
• visual loss can be caused by macula oedema which is extremely difficult to detect ophthalmoscopically—exudates may or may not be present;
• but an unexplained drop in visual acuity of more than one line of Snellen chart which does not correct with the aid of a pin hole should raise the suspicion of maculopathy.

Preproliferative retinopathy (Plate 3, facing page 22)
This is worsening background retinopathy with new, specific features heralding the onset of proliferative retinopathy. Urgent referral is required.
Features include:
• cotton wool spots (soft exudates). Caused by focal retinal infarcts—almost 'fluffy'. A single cotton wool spot is said to be not diagnostic of preproliferative retinopathy but not many general practitioners would take the chance. Refer;
• venous dilatation;
• venous beading—small grape-like or sausage-like dilatations along a large vein;
• venous looping—hard to spot. They are like little hand bag handles usually at the bifurcation of a vein;
• larger haemorrhages—more than half the size of the disc, often with a darker hue.

Proliferative retinopathy (Plate 4, facing page 22)
This is due to increasing retinal ischaemia and develops in up to 50% of IDDM after 20 years of diabetes.
Features include:
• neo-vascularisation. New vessels at the disc or in the periphery. These

look like fine, wiry, wiggly vessels growing chaotically in the retinal plane rather than following the normal branching pattern;
• retinal detachment. The new vessels are attached to the vitreous gel which then detaches from the retina dragging and stretching the new vessels into the space created;
• pre-retinal and vitreous haemorrhages. New vessels can bleed, either into the vitreous or into the space newly created between the vitreous and retina causing complete or partial sudden loss of vision;
• fibrous proliferation. This occurs alongside the new vessels with subsequent cicatrisation, traction and retinal detachment.

So if you see any of these fine, wiggly, new vessels, refer urgently.

A simple scheme to examine the eye
• Test visual acuity regularly (at least annually and more frequently in patients with known retinopathy) using a well lit Snellen chart at the correct distance.
• If refractive error or vision $<\frac{6}{6}$ in either eye re-test using pin hole (see Appendix 2).
• Dilate pupils using 1% tropicamide. (Not if glaucoma.)
• Position ophthalmoscope 50 cm away from patient.
• Check red reflex with scope set at 0 (easy). Then check anterior structures of eye by clicking the dioptre wheel from +20 to 0 on the black numbers (rather difficult).
• Move ophthalmoscope in until retina comes into focus.
• Examine retina; first disc, then nasal quadrants, then temporal quadrants, then lastly macula area. An easy way to find the macula is to ask the patient to look directly at the light.
• Examining with the green light beam helps to show up vessels.

A common confusing finding is the Drusen or colloid body. These look rather like exudates but appear deep seated in the retina and do not have the characteristic 'slapped on' appearance. If you see them on the macula and are not sure, refer. In diabetic retinopathy expect to see microaneurysms and haemorrhages as well.

When to refer — checklist
• Unexplained drop in visual acuity of two lines or more of Snellen chart since last reviewed. (Routine.)
• Background retinopathy and visual acuity worse than $\frac{6}{12}$ not correctable by spectacles or pin hole. (Routine.)
• Ophthalmoscope abnormalities. Maculopathy, preproliferative or proliferative retinopathy. (Urgent.)
• A vitreous or pre-retinal haemorrhage. (Urgent, same day.)

- Any sudden loss of vision. (Urgent, same day.)
- Cannot visualise the retina adequately.

See also:
  Questionnaire, page 83, Retinopathy.

Microalbuminuria

Microalbuminuria is a marker of vascular injury in diabetes and targets those patients who are likely to develop significant problems.

• For IDDM microalbuminuria is an important predictor of nephropathy with up to 80% developing it over the following 10 years compared to only 6% of those without it.

• For NIDDM it predicts progression to nephropathy to a lesser extent.

• Microalbuminuria is a strong predictor of cardiovascular disease in both IDDM and NIDDM.

• It is defined as a urinary albumin excretion rate below the detection limit of standard dipstick methods of between 20 µg/min and 200 µg/min.

• Microalbuminuria is common. It develops in up to 20% of IDDM and 25% of NIDDM.

Screening and diagnosis

• Screen only those dipsticks negative for proteinuria.

• It is detected:

by screening on the first morning urine specimen using either a dipstick test method specific for microalbuminuria

or

by measuring the urinary albumin (in mg) to urinary creatinine (in mmol) ratio on the first morning urine specimen (20 ml of urine in a sterile container with no preservative). A value of >3.5 in women and >2.5 in men is abnormal and correlates with an albumin excretion rate of above 20 µg/minute.

• If albumin:creatinine ratio is raised repeat within 6–12 weeks to confirm.

• Infection at the time of sampling should be excluded.

When and whom to test

• In IDDM from 5 years after diagnosis and then annually up to the age of 65 years.

• In NIDDM the evidence for benefit from screening is not yet clear cut and there is no consensus regarding routine screening (some units in the UK are screening from 6 months after diagnosis).

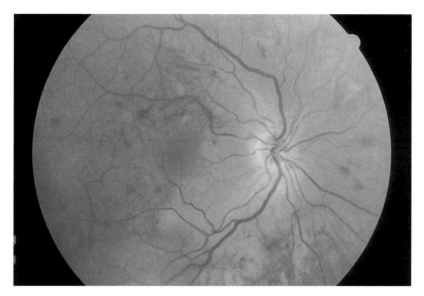

Plate 1 Background retinopathy. Typical microaneurysms (dots) and haemorrhages (blots) are seen throughout the fundus in this patient with extensive background changes.

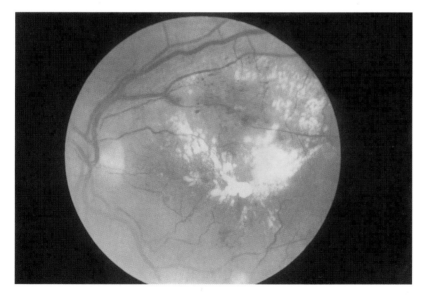

Plate 2 Maculopathy. Large collections of hard exudates in the region of the macula due to vessels leaking serum lipoproteins into the retina (so-called circinate exudates). Visual acuity will be reduced.

[*facing page 22*]

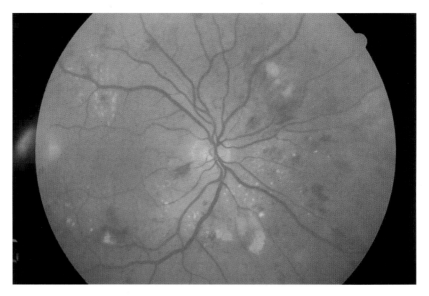

Plate 3 Pre-proliferative retinopathy. Increasing numbers of cotton wool spots (soft exudates) are visible around the retina, due to focal retinal infarcts. This fundus shows also hard exudates and several large haemorrhages.

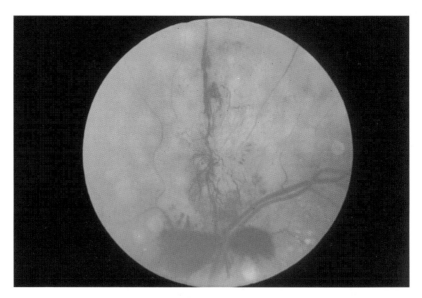

Plate 4 Proliferative retinopathy. A proliferation of fine wiry, wiggly vessels growing chaotically around the optic disc, with two large pre-retinal haemorrhages inferiorly. This patient has been treated with pan-retinal photocoagulation.

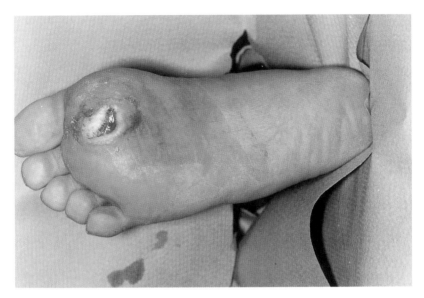

Plate 5 Neuropathic ulcer. Typical 'painless' ulcer located under the heads of the 1st and 2nd metatarsal.

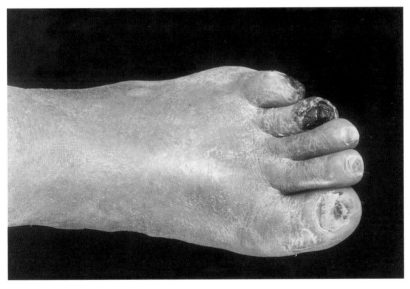

Plate 6 Ischaemic ulcer. Gangrene at the tips of the 4th and 5th toes. Note the dry appearance of the skin due to co-existent neuropathy.

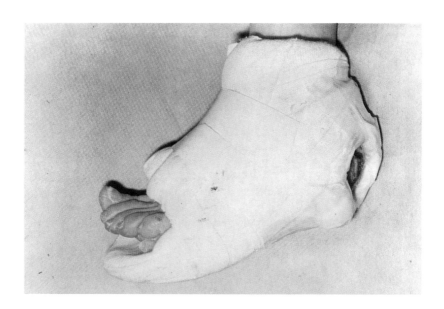

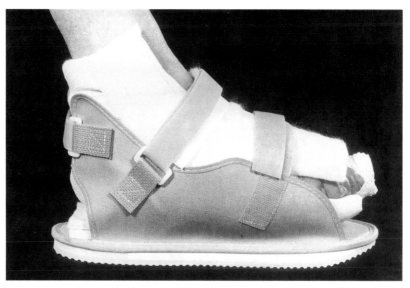

Plates 7 and 8 Scotchcast boot. These lightweight but strong protective boots allow the patient to remain ambulatory and shows a window protecting and relieving pressure at the site of a neuropathic ulcer.

- Screening by standard dipstick methods, although less sensitive, is frequently performed and the finding of trace albuminuria on at least two occasions in the first morning urine specimen should prompt the course of action detailed below.

Management
- Collect midsteam urine specimen to exclude infection and haematuria. Check renal function (U & Es and creatinine).
- Aim for tight glycaemic control. Any improvement will reduce the risk of nephropathy.
- Aim for tight blood pressure control with ACE inhibitors as first choice if no contraindications. A useful target in the UK is <140/90, in USA <130/85.
- Where ACE inhibitors are contraindicated, or where additional blood pressure control is required, consider using an alpha blocker or calcium antagonist.
- Consider using an ACE inhibitor even if normotensive.
- Increase vigilance with regard to screening for other diabetic complications (eyes, lipids, feet and cardiovascular.) Discourage smoking.
- Refer to specialist clinic if any difficulty in achieving target levels of glycaemic or blood presure control.

See also:
   Skill Topic 15, page 33, Hypertension and diabetes.

Diabetic nephropathy

Diabetic nephropathy is characterised by *persistent proteinuria* (dipstick positive for albumin at 1 plus or 0.3 g/l or >200 µg/min on a timed sample) in the presence of an *elevated blood pressure*. Creatinine may be normal in the earlier stages.

Here are a few points:

• Urine should be screened at least annually to detect proteinuria — NIDDM patients from diagnosis, IDDM patients from 5 years after diagnosis until age 65.

• In IDDM nephropathy develops in up to 20–30% of cases. The incidence has been falling in recent decades.

• In NIDDM nephropathy develops in 10% of cases. However, most patients succumb to the ravages of cardiovascular and cerebrovascular injury before it develops.

• In practice, if the patient is persistently Albustix positive (or similar dipstick method for detecting albuminuria) in the presence of retinopathy with no other evidence or history of renal disease, then consider as having nephropathy secondary to diabetes. Very few patients require a renal biopsy to confirm diagnosis.

• It is associated with an increased incidence of retinopathy, neuropathy and cardiovascular problems. (This simply reflects the fact that blood vessel damage is unlikely to be confined to the kidneys.)

• As a typical example of an IDDM patient who subsequently develops nephropathy, the natural history *without intervention* may be like this:

> 5–10 years after diagnosis patient develops microalbuminuria
>
> 5–10 years later patient develops clinical nephropathy (Albustix positive)
>
> 5 years later GFR has fallen to 50% and creatinine starts to rise
>
> 5 years later end stage renal failure occurs.

• Once the creatinine reaches 200 mol/l the progress towards end stage renal failure without effective blood pressure control is relentless and predictable.

• Once nephropathy is established tight glycaemic control does not significantly influence its progression. This contrasts with microalbuminuria where tight control of blood glucose *does* influence the progression towards nephropathy.

However
- Effective blood pressure control (<140/90) is *essential* to slow progression in both the microalbuminuric and nephropathic phases.
- ACE inhibitors should be considered in all patients with microalbuminuria or nephropathy unless contraindicated (see Skill Topic 15, Hypertension).
- Where ACE inhibitors are contraindicated, and tight blood pressure control is required, consider alternative agents such as an alpha blocker or calcium antagonist.

When to refer
- A low threshold for referral is appropriate—most patients with diabetic nephropathy will need specialist supervision.
- If there is proteinuria and any difficulty in achieving target levels of glycaemic or blood pressure control. See Skill Topic 8, Targets for control.
- If proteinuria and creatinine are above normal range.

Remember
Accelerated malignant hypertension can occur in patients with diabetes. If blood pressure is markedly raised with proteinuria and particularly if there are typical flame shaped retinal haemorrhages, consider this possibility rather than putting it down to nephropathy.

Diabetic neuropathy

Diabetic neuropathy is extremely common in diabetes and can lead to significant symptoms and complications. Most patients present with a symmetrical peripheral sensorimotor neuropathy affecting the legs.

Typical somatic diabetic neuropathies

- Chronic distal sensory loss.
  The commonest type seen and usually irreversible. It is often symmetrical with numbness, tingling and/or pain. Muscle wasting of intrinsic foot muscles may be present predisposing to foot deformity. However, there are often no symptoms so need to screen for high risk foot (see Skill Topic 13, Diabetic foot problems).
- Acute painful neuropathy.
  Mainly affects distal lower limbs. Onset during periods of hyperglycaemia, with improving control or at diagnosis. Normally recovers within 6–12 months. Pain is often distressing and described as burning or shooting. Tight glycaemic control and analgesia required.
- Amyotrophy or proximal motor neuropathy.
  Classically affects the thigh leading to pain, weakness and/or wasting with or without sensory loss. Typically absent knee jerk. Can effect buttock also. Important to exclude nerve root compression. Usually resolves within 6–12 months with tight glycaemic control.
- Focal nerve palsy.
  Occasionally leads to an ocular palsy (3rd or 6th).
  If multiple = mononeuritis multiplex. Probably ischaemic in origin and usually recovers in 3–6 months.

Autonomic diabetic neuropathy

Now here's a list to think about:
- Postural hypotension.
- Bladder dysfunction—large atonic bladder.
- Impotence.
- Hypoglycaemia unawareness. This can be related to length of time since diagnosis or be secondary to tight metabolic control with frequent episodes of hypoglycaemia leading to blunting of the counter-regulatory hormonal responses due to a low blood glucose.

- Sweating. Peripheral loss, sometimes with paradoxical upper truncal hyperhydrosis. Often occurs after meals or at night and can be mistaken for hypoglycaemia (known as gustatory sweating).
- Vomiting due to gastric atony.
- Diarrhoea.

Management of diabetic neuropathy
- Exclude other treatable causes such as drugs, alcohol and nerve root lesions.
- Tighten metabolic control. This may require transfer to insulin.

Painful somatic neuropathy
- Simple analgesics such as aspirin or codeine may help relieve pain.
- For pain use simple analgesics first and if no improvement try low dose amitriptyline.
- Other agents which may also be tried for pain include carbamazepine, phenytoin, mexilitine, polyunsaturated oils, etc. Epidurals occasionally of benefit.

Autonomic neuropathy
- Therapy varies according to the presenting symptom.
- For impotence see Skill Topic 19, Erectile dysfunction.
- For postural hypotension check first that there is no other drug cause then consider use of pressure stockings or agents such as non-steroidal anti-inflammatories or fludrocortisone to increase vascular volume.
- For diarrhoea consider anti-spasmodics such as codeine phosphate after exclusion of other organic causes.

See also:
Questionnaire, page 84, Diabetic neuropathy.

Diabetic foot problems

Foot problems in diabetes place a large burden on hospital in-services. Education and self-care are cost effective ways of reducing this distressing complication.

Foot problems are brought about by the triad of:

1 neuropathy;
2 infection;
3 vascular insufficiency.

The clinical picture depends on the relative combinations of these three factors.

Neuropathy

Leads to:

• sensory loss—predisposing to ulcer formation;
• motor weakness of the small foot muscles predisposing to foot deformity;
• autonomic disturbance which causes lack of sweating, increased skin perfusion and dry skin;
• ulcers which develop at points of high pressure, under the tips of the toes, metatarsal heads and heels (Plate 5, facing page 22).

Infection

• Can enter through minor skin lesions or callous.
• Spreads along tissue planes to cause necrosis.
• Can progress to osteomyelitis.

Vascular insufficiency

Can cause:

• typical signs and symptoms of claudication;
• ischaemic ulcers often on the lateral border of foot and tips of toes (Plate 6, facing page 22);
• rapid progression to gangrene.
    In general practice it is important:
• to educate the patient about proper preventative foot care (patient education leaflets are very useful);

- to detect the *high risk foot* and prescribe appropriate footwear to reduce the risk of ulceration breaking out.

The *high risk* foot is typically:

warm, due to autonomic disturbance (unless there is gross vascular insufficiency);

not sweaty (dry, in fact!) due to autonomic neuropathy;

numb, tingly and burning, especially in bed, due to sensory neuropathy;

calloused, due to sensory neuropathy;

misshapen, with claw toes, hallux valgus, prominent metatarsal heads;

poorly shod, in ill-fitting footwear.

A diabetic with a high risk foot should be referred to a multidisciplinary diabetic foot clinic if possible.

Key points
- A patient with neuropathy may not feel the pain of ischaemia.
- An ulcer will not heal in the presence of ischaemia.

To examine the foot in general practice

- *Test* for:
  vibration sense (with a 128c tuning fork placed over the big toe);
  fine touch and pin prick (but fine touch can be preserved until a late stage);
  knee and ankle reflexes.
- *Look* for:
  skin texture (thin?);
  skin sweating (dry?);
  skin colour and capillary return (press your finger into the pulp of the toes and note how long it takes to return to normal pink colour);
  foot shape (see above).
- *Feel* for:
  pulses;
  temperature.
- *Check* for:
  callous and corns;
  ingrowing nails;
  skin breaks (check between toes);
  footwear (appropriate?) rubbing.

Management of diabetic foot problems

• Regular chiropody to remove excessive callous formation and long nails.

• Simple ulcers should be treated with non-adherent dry dressings and saline irrigation.

• Treat infection aggressively (often high dose intravenous antibiotics required).

• Debride and drain deep-seated infection.

• Plantar and heel ulcers will require a pressure relieving technique such as the Scotchcast boot to promote healing (Plates 7 & 8, facing page 22).

• If infection or ulcers are present and pulses are weak arrange a full vascular assessment, including Doppler studies, to exclude ischaemia.

• Early referral to a specialist clinic is the best course of action as infection and ulcers can rapidly progress.

See also:
  Scenario 10
  Questionnaire, page 85, Foot problems.

Large vessel disease and diabetes

Macrovascular injury is common in diabetes, particularly in NIDDM, and accounts for significant morbidity and mortality. Whereas microvascular disease will lead to problems principally affecting the eye and kidney, it is important to recognise that up to 70% of NIDDM and 20–30% of IDDM deaths are due to the combined effects of coronary heart and cerebrovascular disease. Therefore, careful monitoring of patients with either IDDM or NIDDM for large vessel disease is paramount to detect treatable problems at an early stage. Co-existent risk factors should be vigorously addressed including smoking, hypertension, obesity and hyperlipidaemia. Treatment with aspirin should be considered in all patients with macrovascular disease.

Large vessel disease may present as:

1 Ischaemic heart disease.
2 Peripheral vascular disease.
3 Stroke or transient ischaemic attacks.

Ischaemic heart disease

• May present with angina, or in those with autonomic neuropathy with breathlessness alone. Do resting electrocardiograph and consider early referral for exercise stress test.

• Silent ischaemia (i.e. no chest pains) carries the same prognosis as for those presenting with pain.

• Angioplasty and coronary bypass surgery are just as effective in patients with diabetes.

Peripheral vascular disease

• Enquire about intermittent claudication. In the presence of neuropathy the symptoms may be more that of weakness of the limb rather than pain. Examine the leg for proximal and distal pulses and look for signs of ischaemia affecting the toes (see Skill Topic 13, Diabetic foot problems). Consider early referral to a vascular surgeon for Doppler studies (before and after exercise) and possible angiography. Discrete vessel disease may be amenable to angioplasty and diffuse disease to reconstructive bypass.

• Absent pulses on their own, without symptoms or signs of ischaemia, are not a sufficient indication for referral to a vascular surgeon.

Stroke or transient ischaemic attacks

• Patients who make a good recovery from a stroke or who present with transient ischaemic attacks (neurological deficit lasting less than 24 hours) should be investigated with Doppler studies of the carotid and vertebral vessels in order to determine the degree of vessel disease. Carotid endarterectomy is increasingly undertaken when vessel narrowing is greater than 70% in the presence of symptoms.

Hypertension and diabetes

Hypertension accelerates the progression of diabetic complications and there has been a recent trend towards a more aggressive approach to treatment. Blood pressure should be measured after at least 3 minutes rest either supine or sitting using the appropriate sized cuff. All patients should have their blood pressure measured at latest annually and more frequently if borderline.

Therapy should be introduced if after repeated measurements over a 3 month period the blood pressure is consistently raised. Patients with blood pressures >200/105 should be monitored for a shorter period of time.

What level should be treated?

The precise level to which blood pressure should be lowered in diabetes is still uncertain. However, lowering blood pressure is important to reduce the risk of vascular injury and retard the progression of microvascular complications, notably nephropathy. Recommendations vary from country to country but a consensus is beginning to develop as follows.
- For *all* IDDM patients and NIDDM patients with target organ damage: treat if blood pressure is consistently equal to or higher than 140/90.
- For NIDDM patients without target organ damage: treat if blood pressure is consistently equal to or higher than 160/90.

Which agent should be used?

Initial treatment should include lifestyle changes including weight loss, exercise and less alcohol and salt.

IDDM patients
- First choice is an ACE inhibitor particularly if microalbuminuria or proteinuria is present. See Skill Topic 10, Microalbuminuria. In the presence of nephropathy, treatment with an ACE inhibitor should be considered regardless of the level of blood pressure. Even in the presence of microalbuminuria there is evidence that ACE inhibitors confer a beneficial effect in normotensive IDDM patients over and above simple blood pressure control. If ACE inhibitors are contraindicated consider using an alpha blocker (doxazosin). If blood pressure remains elevated a

second or third antihypertensive may need to be added to achieve good blood pressure control.

• Second choice: alpha blocker (doxazosin), calcium antagonist or low dose thiazide.

NIDDM patients

• First choice remains an ACE inhibitor *but* treatment needs to be tailored individually.

Care must be exercised in using ACE inhibitors in NIDDM patients in view of the increased prevalence of macrovascular disease and potential for renal artery stenosis. Renal function should be checked before initiating therapy and most importantly 7–14 days later to make certain there has been no significant deterioration (if creatinine rises by greater than 30% the ACE inhibitor should be stopped and investigations for renal artery stenosis started).

• Second choice: alpha blocker (doxazosin), calcium antagonist or low dose thiazide.

In both IDDM and NIDDM patients

• Patients with co-morbidity such as ischaemic heart disease may benefit from a calcium antagonist or beta blocker.

• Alpha blockers such as doxazosin are helpful in combination with other agents.

• Monitor for other side-effects associated with antihypertensive therapy such as hyperlipidaemia, electrolyte disturbances and erectile dysfunction.

• Refer if unable to achieve target blood pressure.

See also:

Questionnaire, page 85, Hypertension and diabetes.

Hyperlipidaemia and diabetes

Diabetic patients are both more prone to lipid abnormalities and more at risk from their adverse effects than non-diabetic patients, thus accelerating the progression of vascular disease.

Intervention studies with HMG CoA reductase inhibitors have shown convincingly that substantial reductions in mortality and morbidity can be achieved without adverse effects; subgroup analysis has shown this effect to apply equally to diabetic patients with established cardiovascular disease.

There is, however, as yet a paucity of information about the treatment of hyperlipidaemic diabetic patients *without* established cardiovascular disease; further large scale studies are in progress to clarify this important area.

Before treating with drugs

• Exclude secondary causes such as hypothyroidism, excess alcohol, drugs (thiazides and beta blockers commonly), nephropathy.
• Optimise metabolic control (triglycerides and LDL-cholesterol may both improve).
• Encourage lifestyle changes to reduce fat intake, to increase exercise and to stop smoking.

What level should be treated?

• For secondary prevention (patient has cardiovascular disease): cholesterol should be lowerered to <4.8 mmol/l after a myocardial infarction and to <5.5 mmol/l if angina, peripheral vascular disease or carotid artery disease.
• For primary prevention (patient has no cardiovascular disease): less is known. Certain groups of diabetic patients are at particular high risk: those with a low HDL, or with a strong family history of IHD, or with hypertension, or of Indo-Asian origin. For these patients a consensus is emerging that a cholesterol of <6.5 mmol/l is a reasonable target.
• The threshold for intervention in isolated hypertriglyceridaemia is also uncertain. Many guidelines recommend therapy for raised triglyceride

levels above 4.5 mmol/l but lower levels should be treated if there are co-existent risk factors or evidence of vascular disease.

Which drug?

The pattern of lipid abnormality should help you decide which agent to try first. Side-effects are common with all lipid lowering agents and the patient should be carefully monitored.

• If the total cholesterol and LDL-cholesterol are raised and triglycerides are low or normal then try a statin first after checking liver function. Bile acid sequestrants are poorly tolerated and may increase triglycerides.

• If isolated hypertriglyceridaemia then consider using a fibrate or nicotinic acid derivative

• If the total cholesterol, LDL-cholesterol and triglycerides are *all* raised then try a fibrate or atorvastatin first particularly if the HDL cholesterol is low. (This pattern is commonly seen in NIDDM patients.)

• Refer if therapy with a single agent fails.

See also:

Scenario 9

Skill Topic 8, page 16, Targets for control.

Intercurrent illness

Guidelines differ for IDDM and NIDDM and they are therefore considered separately. Patients should be encouraged to make contact with a member of the diabetes team (general practitioner, diabetes specialist nurse or hospital) at an early stage if unwell, are vomiting, have high urine or blood tests or are uncertain about what to do.

Adult IDDM sick days

Remember
- Vomiting can cause ketoacidosis, but diabetic ketoacidosis can cause vomiting.
- During illness insulin requirements usually go up.
- It is never appropriate to reduce insulin during illness even if the patient is eating less; more often an increase of 10–20% is required (unless blood tests are low or urine negative).
- The cardinal signs and symptoms of ketoacidosis are acidotic breathing (air hunger), fruity smell, drowsiness, abdominal pain, nausea, vomiting and dehydration.
- Think of an occult infection, particularly if pyrexial, e.g. silent pneumonia, urinary tract infection or abscess.

In practice
- Patients should be encouraged to test blood glucose 4–6 hourly. Patients using urinalysis only should increase frequency of testing to at least twice daily.
- Patients will probably be anorexic but meals can be substituted by frequent small snacks, e.g. toast and honey, ice cream, muesli bars, fruit, banana milk shakes, dry biscuits, crisps or bland food such as boiled rice, mashed potato.
- If vomiting or diarrhoea:
  If blood glucose >15 mmol/l sip water or diet cola, diet lemonade. Aim for 1 glass (200 ml) per hour
  If blood glucose <15 mmol/l drink sweetened drinks such as flat, ordinary lemonade or cola diluted 50:50 or glucose based drink diluted $\frac{1}{3}:\frac{2}{3}$ with water.

- Test for urinary ketones and if moderate or severe discuss admission with diabetic or on-call medical team.
- Do not be afraid to give extra soluble insulin 6 hourly in addition to the patient's standard regimen. Give 4–6 units if blood glucose >15 mmol/l. Seek advice if blood glucose >20 mmol/l. Patients should be told to ring doctor if blood glucose >15 mmol/l for >24 hours when ill.
- Do not be afraid to ask for help. Diabetes specialist nurses are experienced in managing sick days.

Child IDDM sick days

- Never stop the insulin.
- Basically the same as for adults, giving frequent small volume drinks containing sugar remembering that many infections are clinically undetectable in the early stages.
- Children become dehydrated more rapidly than adults and progression into ketoacidosis is a potential concern.
- Parents of children under 12 years of age are advised to give an extra 2–4 units of quick-acting insulin if blood glucose >20 mmol/l during an illness. Older children/adolescents may have 4–6 units extra.
- If vomiting persists advice must be sought and the child referred to hospital.

Adult NIDDM sick days

Remember
- NIDDM patients can become severely hyperglycaemic during illness.
- NIDDM patients may require a short period of insulin therapy (best done in hospital).
- Although less common than in IDDM ketoacidosis can still occur.

In practice
- Patients can take sugar free, clear fluid and if necessary substitute meals with frequent, small, carbohydrate snacks, e.g. toast, dry biscuits, crisps, breakfast cereal. If vomiting can take dilute lemonade or cola.
- Patients should be told to consult their own doctor if their urine test shows 2% for >24 hours during illness or blood glucose >15 mmol/l.
- Test for urinary ketones and if moderate or severe discuss admission with diabetic or on-call medical team.
- Consider need for short term insulin therapy in hospital if blood glucose >20 mmol/l for >24 hours.

See also:
    Scenario 11
    Questionnaire, page 87, Intercurrent illness.

Hypoglycaemia

For the diabetic patient fear of hypoglycaemia can outweigh concern about the future development of complications. At best, a hypoglycaemic reaction can be an unpleasant mixture of sweating, trembling, weakness and visual disturbance and at worst, a severe episode of seizure or coma requiring hospital admission.

• Always try and confirm with a capillary blood glucose test if unsure whether patient's behaviour is due to hypoglycaemia. Give glucose or other carbohydrate first if unable to test.

• Hypoglycaemia is reported to account for approximately 4% of all deaths of patients with IDDM.

• Not surprisingly, severe hypoglycaemia occurs more commonly in intensively treated patients. The DCCT showed a 3-fold increase in severe episodes (patient required assistance).

• The issue of whether repeated hypoglycaemia can cause permanent cognitive impairment is unresolved although it may be the case in children aged less than 5 years.

• Hypoglycaemia unawareness occurs in up to 25% of IDDM patients. It arises either because of a long length of time since diagnosis (so-called 'duration linked') or because control has been too tight in recent weeks or months. These patients may become biochemically hypoglycaemic but do not experience the usual neuroglycopenic warning symptoms and signs and thus develop confusion or collapse before they are able to take corrective action. For patients with too tight control but not those with 'duration linked' hypoglycaemia unawareness the syndrome may be reversed by running sugar levels a little higher (7–11 mmol/l) and avoiding hypoglycaemia for a period of time, perhaps 4–8 weeks.

• Hypoglycaemia can occur in NIDDM patients on OHAs. If the drugs are of the long-acting type such as glibenclamide or chlorpropramide hypoglycaemia can be prolonged and necessitate hospital admission.

The reader will be familiar with the method of correcting a 'hypo' by injection (glucagon 1 mg i.m. and/or 20–30 ml of dextrose 50% i.v.) but often oral therapy is all that is needed in a conscious and reasonably co-operative patient. Here is a guide as to what and how much should be given.

1 Give rapid-acting carbohydrate first, e.g.
   - 50 ml glucose based drink;
   - 100 ml fizzy drink, e.g. cola, lemonade;
   - 100 ml pure orange juice;
   - 3 glucose tablets;
   - 2 teaspoons sugar, jam or honey.

The above provide 10 g of carbohydrate. Repeat after 5 minutes if no response.

2 Follow up with long-acting carbohydrate, e.g.
   - next meal if due;
   - slice of wholemeal bread;
   - small bowl of cereal;
   - glass of milk and a digestive biscuit.

See also:

Scenario 6

Questionnaire, page 86, Hypoglycaemia.

Erectile dysfunction

Erectile dysfunction in patients with diabetes is extremely common, with up to 50% impotent over the age of 50 years (compared to 15–20% in those without diabetes). The erectile problems vary from difficulty in achieving an erection to difficulty maintaining it long enough for satisfactory intercourse. Several factors contribute to erectile dysfunction including autonomic neuropathy, vascular insufficiency and psychological problems. However, a precise aetiologic diagnosis is not usually required for satisfactory management and unless it is obvious that psychological factors are a dominant feature counselling is not warranted.

Management of erectile dysfunction

• Exclude other treatable hormonal causes such as hyperprolactinaemia and a low testosterone.

• Discuss the various options listed below with his partner present if possible. Give them time to think it over once they have some literature and/or a video.

There are essentially a number of options available:

• Vacuum assist devices. These are effective in up to 70% of patients regardless of the aetiology. A perspex cylinder is placed over the penis and air is pumped out to produce an erection which is maintained by an elastic constriction band. Bruising at the site of the band is the commonest problem with this method.

• Intracavernosal therapy. The patient is taught to inject the prostaglandin alprostadil into the base of the penis to produce the erection by relaxing smooth muscle. Patients are advised to attend casualty or a urology ward for detumescence by aspiration or injection if the erection lasts longer than 4 hours.

• Intraurethral administration of alprostadil. This is a new system which is increasingly being used. The patient is taught to insert a small pellet containing alprostadil using an applicator into the urethra where it dissolves. Success rates up to 70% have been reported.

• Oral agents. Sildenafil is a novel oral treatment for erectile dysfunction. The process of an erection involves the release of nitric oxide into the corpus cavernosum during sexual stimulation. Nitric oxide activates an enzyme called guanylate cyclase, which increases cyclic guanosine monophosphate (cGMP). cGMP induces smooth muscle relaxation in the corpus cavernosum allowing blood to flow into the penis. Sildenafil enhances this effect by inhibiting a specific phosphodiesterase involved in the breakdown of cGMP in the corpus cavernosum. Success rates of 60–70% have been reported.

• Finally, for those who do not relish self-injection or vacuum devices tubes then a penile prosthesis implant may be considered. This can range from the simple insertion of flexible rods into the corpus cavernosum on each side to more sophisticated devices which allow the man to pump up the erection as required. Patients need to be highly selected for these procedures and should receive counselling.

Key point

Remember to ask your male patients with diabetes if they are experiencing erectile problems. Only the patient should be forgiven for being embarrassed — not the doctor or nurse!

Diabetes in Indo-Asians

There is a high prevalence of diabetes in the Indo-Asian communities of the UK which increases with age to over 20% in those aged 65 years compared to 8% in the indigenous population. Many of the microvascular and macrovascular complications are higher also. There is controversy as to the cause of these high rates; genetic predisposition, obesity, insulin resistance, diet and environment have all been cited as possible factors.

Which type of diabetes?

The majority of patients develop NIDDM with many eventually progressing to insulin due to OHA failure. The incidence of IDDM is reported as lower.

Complications

High rates of coronary heart disease are reported even though levels of cholesterol, blood pressure or smoking have not been shown to be different from those in the indigenous white population. Microvascular complication rates are similar except for nephropathy where the rates are several-fold higher.

Management of diabetes in Indo-Asians

• Diets are traditionally high in saturated fats and rapidly absorbed carbohydrates. Patients should be advised to use less animal derived oils such as ghee and to grill more often. Desserts are typically very sweet and should be avoided. A dietician sensitive to their culture is often the best person to offer advice.

• Weight reduction is important. Obesity is often viewed as implying well-being and wealth. Exercise should be encouraged.

• Insulin therapy should be introduced once OHAs have failed. Many patients often prove to be insulin resistant and require larger doses of insulin. The combined use of metformin and insulin in these patients occasionally proves beneficial.

• Avoid animal insulins in patients who do not want porcine or bovine insulin for religious reasons. Always inform the patient of the type of insulin you are about to prescribe.

- Screen for complications regularly and check for co-existent vascular risk factors.
- Fasting for Ramadan poses problems mainly for patients on insulin as during this period no food or water is permitted during the day from sunrise to sunset. Although patients on insulin are not expected to fast many do so. As the total amount of food consumed over the fasting period is usually less than normal despite a large meal before sunrise and at the end of the fast, a reduction of each insulin dose of 10–20% is advised. It is important that patients should remain on twice daily insulin and not omit any doses. NIDDM patients on sulphonylureas are best advised to take short-acting preparations such as tolbutamide or gliclazide before the morning and evening meals without a daytime dose.

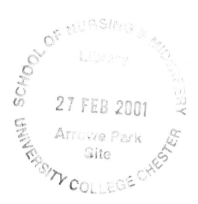

Pregnancy

Perinatal mortality (number of deaths from 28 weeks onwards to the end of the first week of life per 1000 births) due to maternal diabetes has fallen markedly over the last two decades from around 20–30% in the 1950s to less than 2% in recent times in Leicester and other centres due to a combination of factors including tighter control at conception and during pregnancy, combined obstetric and diabetes clinics, regular review throughout pregnancy and regular screening to assess growth and possible complications.

There are three groups of patients to consider.

1 Those who have established IDDM.

2 Those who develop diabetes in pregnancy (gestational diabetes).

3 Those with NIDDM.

Management of established diabetes

• It is essential to plan the pregnancy with tight control *before* conception. Congenital malformations affecting the heart or nervous system are still an important cause of perinatal mortality and thought to relate to poor control at the time of conception and during the first 8 weeks of pregnancy. Many diabetics achieve tight control too late in the pregnancy to avoid problems during organogenesis. Patients should start folic acid (0.4 mg) before conception to lessen the risk of neural tube defects.

• Early consultant referral is essential for assessment (by phone to antenatal clinic).

• Be aware of increased incidence of microvascular complications in pregnancy particularly if control poor.

• Aim for usual weight gain (<12 kg) if possible. If the woman is obese it is unwise to encourage weight reduction as the fetus requires calories for normal neurological development.

• Strict glycaemic control helps to prevent both maternal and fetal complications (particularly fetal macrosomia). Aim for fasting and preprandial levels of <6 mmol/l and postprandial levels <8 mmol/l and HbA1 in the normal range. Hypoglycaemia is more common in pregnancy and patients should be supplied with glucagon and Hypostop.

• Insulin requirements increase substantially in the second half of pregnancy to a mean of about twice the pre-pregnancy dose.

- Regular review by the combined antenatal/diabetes team is of utmost importance.
- The delivery should be planned and timed to occur around 38–39 weeks to lessen the risk of intrauterine death (however, some centres accept this risk and allow the pregnancy to go to 40 weeks and beyond).

Gestational diabetes mellitus

- Defined as diabetes initially detected during pregnancy (usually second trimester) which resolves after delivery.
- The following pregnant women should be screened for gestational diabetes at 28 weeks by performing a glucose tolerance test. The criteria for diagnosis are lower than outside pregnancy. Patients with a 2 hour glucose of >7.8 mmol/l should be considered as having gestational diabetes.

  Obesity >85 kg (in Asians >75 kg).

  Excessive weight gain during current pregnancy.

  Fetal macrosomia or hydramnios.

  Any glycosuria in first trimester.

  Glycosuria on two occasions in second trimester.

  Previous large baby (>4 kg).

  Previous unexplained stillbirth.

  Previous gestational diabetes.

  Family history of diabetes in first degree relatives.

- Gestational diabetes is initially managed by diet alone but if post-prandial blood glucose levels are persistently >8 mmol/l insulin is indicated.
- It is usual for patients with gestational diabetes to have a post-natal glucose tolerance test at 6–8 weeks with hospital review to determine whether the abnormal glucose tolerance has resolved.
- The pregnancy is allowed to proceed to term in most cases.
- Up to 50% of patients with gestational diabetes subsequently develop diabetes during the next 10–20 years.

NIDDM

- It is usual to transfer patients on oral agents to insulin before conception due to the potential risk of teratogenicity and the need to obtain tight glycaemic control. The pregnancy is managed in the same manner as in established IDDM patients.

See also:

Scenario 12

Diabetes in children

- Children with diabetes are managed by a multidisciplinary specialist team.
- Shared care is not appropriate for childhood diabetes but general practitioners should be aware of the correct management of intercurrent infections and hypoglycaemic crises as well as the psychological stress families are under in coping with the difficult problems of achieving adequate control without hypoglycaemia and later in dealing with teenage rebellion.
- The clinical features at diagnosis are usually classical with polyuria, polydipsia, nocturia, enuresis and weight loss. A significant proportion of children, however, present atypically with symptoms such as vomiting, abdominal pain, dehydration, tachypnoea or disturbed consciousness.

> **Key point**
> It is important that when children are found to have significant glycosuria (and hyperglycaemia) they should be referred the same day by telephone because diabetic ketoacidosis can supervene rapidly.

- Home management of newly diagnosed children is nearly always to be preferred, unless hospital admission is required for correction of severe ketoacidosis. This must be co-ordinated by the on-call diabetologist or paediatrician (in Leicester 70% of children are managed in this way).
- Eating disorders are common in young adolescent females who learn to manipulate their diabetes to control their weight (often verging on ketoacidosis).
- Adolescence is a difficult time for all and even if control and attendance is poor it is important to try and keep some form of contact, even if infrequent.

Travel and exercise

Travel

Travelling overseas can be a daunting task for a patient with diabetes on insulin. Careful preparation is required and the airline and insurance company should be warned in advance.

What advice should be given?
• On the day of travel reduce insulin dose by about 10–15% as there is usually a lot of excitement and energy expended. It is reasonable for the blood glucose to run a little higher for the period of travelling in order to avoid hypoglycaemia.
• Advise the patient to carry plenty of carbohydrate to supplement their meals if necessary.
• Monitor diabetes control regularly.
• Travelling across time zones may present a problem if the time difference is greater than 4 hours. On the day of travel patients should take their insulin at the normal time if possible and 'live British Time' for the duration of the flight. On arrival if travelling west to east (time gained) then a small dose of short-acting insulin (perhaps 4–10 units) can be taken before any extra meals (such as an extra lunch). A usual or slightly reduced dose of their normal insulin(s) can then be taken before their evening meal. The following day they should return to their usual regimen.
• Travelling the opposite way (east to west) means that time is lost. Extra soluble insulin can be taken before any extra meals before returning to their usual regimen.
• Each journey should be planned with knowledge of the flight times and time zone differences.

Exercise

Exercise has great potential benefits for diabetic patients. It can:
• reduce blood pressure, weight and lipids;
• increase insulin sensitivity.
However, there are some important points to note:
• Regular, moderate exercise 3–5 times per week for a minimum of 30 minutes is the ideal.

• An exercise session of longer than 20 minutes is likely to need a top-up of quick-acting carbohydrate such as glucose tablets, sugary drinks, pure fruit juice or a chocolate snack bar. The increase in insulin sensitivity which follows exercise may cause delayed hypoglycaemia so it is important to have a snack or meal high in slow-acting complex carbohydrate after the exercise session.

• Regular exercisers may prefer to reduce the prior insulin dose but this must be accompanied by careful SBGM.

Audit

Audit
- Can be a powerful incentive to improve diabetic care.
- Allows health professionals to compare with colleagues the sort of care provided.
- Can facilitate the setting up of district diabetes registers, useful for co-ordinating diabetic services, targeting resources, comparing standards between providers and identifying non-attenders and vulnerable groups.
- Works better if criteria standards are discussed and set at practice or local level.

What is audited?
- You choose!
- Questions you may want answered:
  Is the practice diabetic register complete/up to date?
  Have the 'diabetics' been properly diagnosed?
  How is their metabolic control?
  Are sufficient attempts made to chase defaulters?
  Are patients getting a regular complication screen?
  Are newly diagnosed diabetics managed according to a protocol?
  etc.

Ideally, having identified and quantified a problem area, take action to ameliorate it and then re-audit.

The DCCT has helped to establish 'gold standard' targets for diabetic control which in practice can be difficult to achieve. Whilst individual patients need to be aware of the desirability of achieving as good bio-chemical control as possible, general practitioners looking after cohorts of patients will need to adopt a realistic step by step approach.

(An audit protocol can be obtained from the National Clinical Audit Centre, Department of General Practice, Leicester General Hospital, Leicester LE5 4PW.)

Social factors

Driving

The medical team has a duty to advise diabetic patients about their responsibilities with regard to driving.

- Diet controlled patients need not notify the Driving and Vehicle Licensing Agency (DVLA) unless there is impaired vision.
- All diabetics on insulin or tablets must by law notify DVLA and their insurance company. A change of treatment from tablets to insulin or a significant deterioration in condition would necessitate re-notification.
- Newly treated insulin dependent patients should not drive until stabilised.
- Insulin treated patients must be able to recognise hypoglycaemia and know how to treat it. Some form of 'hypostopper' (see page 41) must be carried at all times in the car and special attention should be made to eating regular meals and snacks whilst driving. Diabetic patients and their doctors may be surprised to learn that insulin is regarded as a drug by the Road Traffic Act and failure to take either suitable preventative or treatment measures for hypoglycaemia may render the patient liable to be charged with the offence of driving under the influence of drugs.
- Insulin treated patients are barred from holding an HGV or PSV licence unless they held such a licence, and were insulin treated, prior to August 1991. From 1997 this restriction includes the driving of goods vehicles of greater than 3.5 tons and larger minibuses of more than 16 seats.
- For a fuller account consult the appropriate chapter in *Medical Aspects of Fitness to Drive* (a book which should be on the shelf of every health professional looking after diabetic patients). See Appendix 5.
- Driving must cease if hypoglycaemia is frequent or there is loss of awareness.

Employment

- Diabetic patients are barred from a career in the Armed Forces, as a civil aviation pilot or in the Police Force.
- Other jobs with a high risk component such as building, working at heights or operating heavy machinery need to be individually assessed by

a diabetes specialist with the patient's clinical condition taken into account.

• The BDA is skilled at providing advice on insurance and occupational pensions.

• Diabetic patients are entitled to register as disabled for employment purposes with access to a Disablement Resettlement Officer based at a Job Centre. In practice, this is only of benefit if there is difficulty in finding work.

• Employers may sometimes harbour unjustified fears about employing diabetic patients and a supporting letter from their general practitioner or specialist can be helpful.

• Employers have a right to dismiss an employee who is medically unfit for the job but the decision must be justified and can be subjected to legal appeal.

• A common misconception is that 'you can't be sacked whilst you're on the sick'. You can, subject to contract and the Disability Discrimination Act.

• Unpredictable late working can cause problems if it cuts across normal meal and injection times. Employers need to be aware that when a diabetic employee sends out for sandwiches it is motivated by necessity not greed!

• The problems of shift working can be overcome by a competent patient particularly if a multiple injection regimen is used. Specialist help is advisable.

• Employers can be reassured that diabetic patients are good employees. The rigours and demands of diabetic life can develop in them a particular maturity and responsibility not necessarily seen in their healthy colleagues.

CLINICAL
SCENARIOS

Initial management

Mr White is a 34 year old Caucasian who has felt unwell for 2 weeks with increasing lethargy and thirst. He thinks he has lost weight and now weighs 68 kg for a height of 175 cm (BMI is 22). Clinical examination is normal. His 36 year old brother has been an insulin dependent diabetic for 12 years.

Urine testing reveals 2% glycosuria with + ketonuria. Venous plasma glucose is 18.2 mmol/l.

Questions

1 Would you hospitalise?

2 What, if any, treatment should be given?

3 What factors in the above history help you to decide whether Mr White has IDDM or NIDDM?

Discussion

1 Hospitalisation is not indicated in this case but he should be referred by phone, the same day. Outpatient management encourages greater patient autonomy from the start.

2 Insulin administered twice daily. A combination of pre-mixed insulins would be suitable.

3 The distinction between IDDM or NIDDM is not always clear cut but the weight loss is the key factor here. In addition the patient's age, the acute onset, the mild ketonuria and the presence of IDDM in a sibling are important pointers towards IDDM.

Consider the following lists:

IDDM	NIDDM
Peak incidence 10–30 years	Peak incidence >40 years
Onset usually acute	Gradual onset
Usually non-obese	Often obese
Ketosis prone	Non-ketotic
Strong family history in siblings	Strong family history
Insulin deficient	Insulin resistance

See also:
Skill Topics 2 and 3, Initial management.
Questionnaire, page 80.

Initial management

Mrs Black is aged 45 and presents with polyuria and polydipsia. She denies weight loss and is eating normally. The notes reveal that she has attended twice in the past 6 months with vaginal thrush. Her 78 year old mother has diabetes for which she takes tablets.

- Her weight is 82 kg for a height of 162 cm.
- Clinical examination is normal.
- Urinalysis reveals 5% glycosuria with no ketones.
- Her blood glucose is 26 mmol/l.

Questions

1 What type of diabetes mellitus is Mrs Black likely to have? List the reasons for your decision.
2 What, if any, treatment would you give?
3 When would you wish to review her?

Discussion

1 Mrs Black has NIDDM. She is obese with a subacute history, no weight loss or ketonuria and a positive family history of NIDDM.

2 Although symptomatic with a high plasma glucose a weight reducing diabetic diet should be tried for 12 weeks. The dietary changes required should be discussed with a dietician.

3 She should be reviewed in 1 week to check symptoms, blood glucose and urine for ketones. If there is no improvement in her symptoms and fasting blood glucose remains above 15 mmol/l then a small dose of an OHA should be started. In this case metformin would be advised in view of her obesity (see Skill Topic 6, Starting oral hypoglycaemic agents). There is room for flexibility; if symptoms are mild, diet therapy could be continued for up to 12 weeks.

At, or soon after, diagnosis she should have her U & Es and lipids checked and should be checked for any sign of microvascular or macrovascular complications.

See also:

Skill Topic 2, Initial management step by step.
Skill Topic 3, Initial management flow chart.

Devise a patient education checklist

Your practice has decided to try and improve the management of newly diagnosed diabetes.

Devise a patient education checklist, for use by the practice nurse, to cover those aspects of diabetes relevant to the newly diagnosed patient. Assume that initial treatment and investigations have been decided. Append two smaller additional checklists for patients on insulin or OHAs.

Checklist
- Simple explanation of diabetes.
- Basic dietary advice (pending dietician appointment).
- Where care will be provided and how often.
- Principles and rationale of diabetic control.
- Recognising a 'hypo' and what to do.
- Urine testing.
- Blood testing (if preferred).
- Simple sickness rules.
- Foot care.
- Exercise.
- Alcohol.
- Smoking.
- Driving.
- Employment.
- BDA.
- Free prescriptions (if on treatment).
- Free eye tests.

Insulin
- Types of insulin.
- Types of syringes (inc. pens).
- How to draw up.
- How to mix insulins.
- Storage and re-use.
- Needle clipper.
- Injection technique.

- Site rotation.
- Adjustment of insulin dose.
- Snacks.

Oral hypoglycaemic agents
- Mode of action (not magic cure).
- Possible side-effects.
- May need increasing.

Poor control and unwell 5 months after diagnosis

Mrs Draper is aged 61 and presents with a 3 month history of a dry mouth and tiredness. She has hypercholesterolaemia. Urine testing reveals glycosuria+++ with no ketones. Blood glucose is 31.2 mmol/l. Her weight is 79 kg, a loss of 3 kg since last weighed 1 year ago, but she thinks that this may be due to her low fat diet. She is commenced on tolbutamide 500 mg thrice daily and further dietary advice is given. Her random blood sugar falls to around 17 mmol/l and after 3 months her HbA1 is 10.9%. However, 5 months after diagnosis she still has blood glucose levels ranging from 10 to 20 mmol/l and her weight has dropped to 65 kg.

Apart from lethargy, there are no other striking features in the history or examination. Thyroid function and plasma viscosity are normal.

Questions

1 What should be the next management step?
2 Comment on the initial management of this case. (You may find it useful to consult Skill Topic 3, page 7, Initial management flow chart.)

Discussion

1 The patient is continuing to lose weight at an excessive rate due to poor glycaemic control. A reasonable weight loss for a woman is 0.5 kg/week (up to 1 kg/week may be expected for the more obese). Although she is not ketotic she now requires insulin and is started on an isosphane insulin twice daily.
2 The decision to manage the patient initially without insulin was justified despite the high presenting glucose — she was not ketotic and there was only a dubious small weight loss.

However, three specific criticisms can be made of the management:
1 As a general rule it is not good practice to start OHAs without at least a short trial of diet. If you feel that the blood glucose needs to be lowered this quickly you should probably be consulting a diabetologist to discuss whether insulin is required.
2 Monitoring the patient's progress by random blood glucose measurements is of limited value; a fasting blood glucose 1 week after diagnosis

and subsequently fortnightly would have given an earlier indication of her need for insulin.

3 At diagnosis the patient's height should be measured so that a BMI can be calculated. This is essential data for deciding which OHA to start. Metformin is the drug of choice for obese patients.

See also:

 Skill Topic 3, Initial management flow chart.

Confusing test results in an IDDM patient

Mr Topping is aged 39 and works as a refuse collector. He has been diabetic for 20 years. His current insulin dose is 25 units of isophane with 10 units of soluble insulin morning and evening. His weight is 68 kg.

At diabetic review he has an HbA1 of 12% although his occasional SBGM (without a meter) are always less than 9 mmol/l. He denies hypoglycaemia, which he makes efforts to avoid whilst at work by eating chocolate snack bars. He mentions also that he has recently had a headache some mornings and has been suffering from nightmares.

Questions

1 What are the possible explanations of his test results and symptoms?
2 What action might you take?

Discussion

1 There is a discrepancy between his HbA1 and home blood glucose results. In the absence of severe uraemia or a haemoglobinopathy, both of which can give a false high HbA1, it is likely that his results are giving a falsely reassuring picture. Possible causes for this are:

- Poor technique or impaired vision.
- Faulty meter (if used) or poorly calibrated.
- Testing at same time every day or when he feels low.
- Fictitious results.

Also of importance is that his total insulin dosage exceeds 1 unit/kg/day and there is therefore a possibility that he is overtreated with insulin, leading to nocturnal hypoglycaemia and rebound morning hyperglycaemia. The morning headache and nightmares could be explained by hypoglycaemia.

Being understandably keen to avoid hypoglycaemia at work, it is also possible that he is overcompensating with daytime snacks. Insulin adjustments in a case like this are likely to require specialist team assistance but it is useful to know that not every IDDM patient with high HbA1 requires an automatic increase in insulin.

Remember also that there may be a second pathology causing poor control—diabetics get thyroid disease too!

2 Mr Topping is likely to need:
- An education session revising his SBGM technique.
- Encouragement to perform SBGM at least twice daily, preferably at different times and an explanation of the rationale of good control. Ask him to check his 3 a.m. blood glucose on a few occasions as it may reveal nocturnal hypoglycaemia.
- A reduction in his evening isophane dose.
- Diet review and 'snack' advice.

See also:
Appendix 1 on the DCCT.
Skill Topic 8, Targets for control.
Questionnaire, pages 81–82.

Unwell elderly diabetic woman

Mrs Jolly is an 83-year-old widow who has diet controlled NIDDM. Following an admission to hospital for an episode of cardiac failure she is started on glibenclamide 5 mg daily. Five months after discharge her HbA1 is quite satisfactory (7.4%) but a month later due to increasing frailty she is taken to live at her daughter's house. Keen to do her best her daughter consults with the dietician and a low fat, sugar reduced diet is started.

Two months later you are called to see Mrs Jolly. Her walking has deteriorated and she is intermittently confused.

Question

What is the most likely diabetes related cause of her symptoms and how could it have been avoided?

Discussion

Hypoglycaemia. The dietary crackdown imposed by the daughter unfortunately precipitated chronic debilitating hypoglycaemia which in fact only became apparent when the patient had an episode of frank collapse. She made a miraculous recovery with intravenous glucose. She should not have been prescribed glibenclamide in the first place as this is a powerful and long-acting drug which achieves most of its hypoglycaemic effect at the lower doses and is unsuitable for use in the elderly. Tolbutamide starting with a low dose would have been a better choice if an OHA was to be used at all.

See also:
   Skill Topic 18.
   Questionnaire page 86, Hypoglycaemia.

Poor control on oral hypoglycaemic agents

Mr Lucas is a 61-year-old sheet metal worker who presents with classical symptoms, a venous plasma blood glucose of 21 mmol/l and no ketones. His weight is steady at 72 kg (BMI is 24) He is started on a diabetic diet which he adheres to strictly. His symptoms settle in 4 weeks and at the 12 week review his fasting blood glucose is 13 mmol/l. He has expressed great fears that the doctors may wish to start him on insulin.

He is started on tolbutamide which is increased to 2 g daily but his control remains poor with a fasting blood glucose of 12.5 mmol/l and HbA1 of 10.1% after a further 3 months. His weight has fallen to 66 kg.

Question
What would be your next step and why?

Discussion
Mr Lucas is now asymptomatic and his weight loss of 6 kg in 6 months is not excessive. His BMI was at the upper limit of the normal range so a gentle weight reducing diet was still appropriate to try and decrease any insulin resistance. His fasting blood glucose remains markedly high despite tolbutamide and therefore metformin should now be added (after checking his renal and liver function and alcohol intake).

Alas, the chances that a biguanide will satisfactorily improve his control are small. His fasting blood glucose was high at 13 mmol/l after the trial of diet and remained virtually the same despite a sulphonylurea. This suggests poor endogenous insulin reserves and that Mr Lucas will be one of the 35% of NIDDM patients who fail to have adequate control after starting OHAs. His aversion to insulin therapy is common and understandable. It may be better for all avenues to be explored before starting insulin, which he may accept initially on a trial basis. He should be reviewed in 2–3 months to assess progress.

See also:
   Skill Topic 5, Oral hypoglycaemic agents.
   Skill Topic 7, Insulin therapy.

Problems of the poorly motivated patient

Mr Brown is a 52-year-old NIDDM patient who is on maximal oral therapy. He is obese at 108 kg and is non-compliant with diet, despite the persuasions of his general practitioner, practice nurse and dietician. He admits to drinking 2 pints of beer per day but probably more on darts night. He has a sedentary factory job. As he often arrives home quite late from the pub he and his wife have taken to sleeping in separate bedrooms.

After a number of grossly elevated HbA1 readings spread over 18 months he reluctantly agrees to twice daily insulin. Unfortunately his weight increases further and his insulin requirements rapidly rise to 120 units per day. His HbA1 is only slightly improved.

Question

Could anything else have been done to improve his management?

Discussion

This case illustrates the difficulties of treating poorly motivated patients and shows how diabetes management can only work as a negotiated and collaborative exercise between the patient and health care team. Unfortunately, although this patient had cordial relations with his practice team, motivation was poor. General practitioners are well placed to understand the patient's psychosocial pressures and a victim blaming approach is of course inappropriate. The decision to start insulin was correct although the outcome was not as good as had been hoped.

Some patients respond well to group education sessions.

The possibility of impotence should be broached directly but with tact—he would probably be unaware of the sort of help now available.

Combining metformin or acarbose with insulin is an increasingly used regimen which may improve metabolic control by decreasing both appetite and insulin resistance.

Formal review of diet by a dietician is advisable for all obese NIDDM patients starting on insulin.

See also:
  Skill Topic 7, Insulin therapy.
  Skill Topic 19, Erectile dysfunction.

As a discussion point, think in general terms about factors in the patient's life which sway his/her motivation and compliance.

Hyperlipidaemia in a 64-year-old diabetic woman

Mrs Grey is aged 64 with acceptably controlled NIDDM on tolbutamide. Her recent fasting blood glucose was 8.7 mmol/l and her HbA1 10.2%. Her serum cholesterol is 6.9 mmol/l, triglycerides 3.1 mmol/l and HDL 0.88 mmol/l. Her blood pressure is 175/90 and her weight is 79 kg.

Question

What action would you take?

Discussion

Mrs Grey has the typical clustering of risk factors for coronary heart disease seen in NIDDM patients: diabetes, hypertension, obesity, moderate hypercholesterolaemia, hypertriglyceridaemia and low HDL. At least she doesn't smoke! The first step is to encourage lifestyle changes. Weight loss, reduced saturated fat in diet, reduced salt, increased exercise and stress reduction could all help to reduce these risk factors.

If these fail then pharmacological intervention is necessary.

• There is room for improvement in diabetic control. Add metformin up to maximum dose (check kidney and liver function first).

• Treat blood pressure. Lipid neutral drugs such as an ACE inhibitor, a calcium antagonist or an alpha blocker are a sensible first choice.

• The treatment of this level of hypercholesterolaemia remains a contentious issue which is currently under examination by on-going clinical trials. Most experts (but not all) would consider that she definitely falls into a treatment category as her cholesterol is >6.5 mmol/l, she is diabetic and her cholesterol : HDL ratio is >5 : 1. It would certainly be worth checking thyroid and renal function. If treated a fibrate or atorvastatin would be a good first choice.

See also:

Skill Topic 15, Hypertension and diabetes.
Skill Topic 16, Hyperlipidaemia and diabetes.
Questionnaire, pages 85–86.

Foot problems

Mr Green is aged 46 and has had diabetes for 10 years. He has poor control on glibenclamide 15 mg daily and metformin 850 mg twice daily. Having defaulted from diabetic follow up for 1 year he attends normal surgery and is found to have retinopathy comprising circinate exudates. He is referred urgently to an eye clinic where preproliferative retinopathy is recorded.

He is changed over to twice daily insulin.

He subsequently presents with an acutely swollen right foot which although painless, is warm and erythematous. Both feet are flat with dropped longitudinal arches. There is reduced sensation below ankle level. He is apyrexial.

Questions
1 What are the possible diagnoses?
2 What action is necessary?

Discussion
Despite the lack of fever, cellulitis should be considered and therefore same-day hospital referral is indicated. The differential diagnosis includes Charcot arthropathy and gout.

Diabetic neuropathy is an important cause of Charcot arthropathy principally affecting the ankle and foot. Neuropathy leads to sensory loss which in turn predisposes to repeated minor trauma causing destructive and hypertrophic changes. The clinical picture is of a warm, swollen foot with erythema. Bone scans and x-rays are useful. This unpleasant complication can be prevented or delayed by screening for the 'high risk foot' when the patient attends for routine review.

See also:
Skill Topic 12, Neuropathy.
Skill Topic 13, Diabetic foot problems.
Questionnaire, pages 84–85.

Treating intercurrent illness

Mrs Jones is a 74-year-old resident of a nursing home. She is an insulin treated NIDDM patient on twice daily isophane insulin. She has had several strokes, is catheterised and is wheelchair bound. Matron rings you at 8.35 p.m. just as you have returned from your evening visits. Apparently Mrs Jones has been off colour all day and is now found to be feverish and to have offensive smelling urine. You ask for her temperature to be taken, for the urine to be tested for sugar and ketones and for a random capillary blood glucose to be measured. You place your supper in the microwave.

Matron phones back the results. Her temperature is 37.6°C, urine shows 5% glycosuria, ketones +, haematuria +, and blood glucose is 28 mmol/l. When you visit the patient you are told that she has just vomited.

Mrs Jones shakes her head and bursts into tears when you mention hospital so you decide to manage the case yourself.

Question
How?

Discussion
• Her urinary tract infection can be managed along the usual lines.
• Capillary blood glucose should be checked every 6 hours. Extra soluble insulin is required and can be given over and above her normal insulin. If you do not have any soluble insulin an emergency chemist will provide it (you should have some in your surgery fridge).
• As the patient improves it will be possible to stop the extra soluble insulin supplements and manage with a simple 10–20% increase in isophane dosage. This allows for a reduction in blood glucose monitoring also.
• Fluid replacement is as per Skill Topic 17, Intercurrent Illness.
• The urine should be checked every 6 hours for ketones. One + (small) is acceptable, if moderate or heavy admission to hospital should be reconsidered.
• If clinical condition deteriorates reconsider hospital admission.

See also:
 Skill Topic 17, Intercurrent illness.
 Questionnaire page 87.

Preconceptual counselling

Mrs Tester is aged 24 and has had IDDM for 13 years. She has had a miscarriage 2 months previously and was told at the hospital that this might not have happened if her glycaemic control had been better. She has heard that miscarriages occur because the baby is malformed and wants to know how likely she is to give birth to a normal child. She also asks how likely it is that her children will develop diabetes.

Question
What would you advise?

Discussion
The average perinatal mortality rate for diabetic pregnancies is approximately 5.0% (many centres have better figures especially if there is a combined obstetric/diabetes service) compared to 0.8% for non-diabetic pregnancies. The rate varies depending on the quality of glycaemic control.

Congenital malformations are estimated to account for about one half of the perinatal mortality in the children of diabetic women.

The chances of a diabetic woman giving birth to a child with a congenital malformation (including non-fatal ones) is 7%, about three times the rate in the general population. Metabolic control at or around the time of conception correlates with the rate of congenital malformations.

There is about a 1 in 40 chance that any child of hers will have diabetes. If the patient with diabetes was the father the risk is around 1 in 20.

Key points
- Glycaemic control needs to be as good as possible early in the pre-pregnancy phase to minimise congenital malformations.
- Glycaemic control throughout pregnancy needs to be as good as possible to optimise the baby's condition at birth and prevent maternal complications such as retinopathy, nephropathy and eclampsia.

See also:
Skill Topic 21, Pregnancy.

Organisation of a general practice diabetic clinic

The senior partner in your practice, Dr Driver, is Chairman of the Anglo-Bermudan Medical Society. Following a recent highly successful educational visit to Bermuda he announces that he has invited a party of Bermudan doctors to your practice for the day. They are particularly keen to see how your diabetic clinic is organised.

Draw up two separate lists of tasks performed by firstly the practice nurse and secondly the general practitioner in your diabetic clinic. Include blood tests and how often they should be performed.

Practice nurse
Checks smoking habit.
Records well-being (? hypos).
Records drugs.
Examines for foot problems.
Measures weight and compares with target weight.
Checks peripheral pulses.
Checks sensation to touch, vibration and pin prick.
Measures blood pressure.
Checks urine for sugar and protein.
Sends off urine test for microalbuminuria (if indicated).
Examines injection sites.
Checks visual acuity ± pin hole.
Dilates pupils.
Takes blood for HbA1 — preferably 6 monthly.
U & Es
Creatinine } yearly (unless more frequent testing indicated).
Lipids

Doctor
Checks medication and changes if necessary.
Checks previous results done in surgery.
Reviews diet, alcohol consumption and smoking habit.
Reviews patient's home urinalysis or SBGM.
Reviews any abnormal findings.
Checks lens for cataracts and fundi (via dilated pupils).

There should be flexibility in how the tasks are divided between doctors and nurses, the above is for guidance only.

The BDA document 'Recommendations for the management of diabetes in primary care' provides further useful information on this subject.

SELF-ASSESSMENT QUESTIONNAIRE

This section is designed primarily as a learning exercise and as a stimulus to refer to other sections of the book. The statements should be answered 'true' or 'false'. There is an intentional omission of a 'do not know' option so that you will be encouraged to attempt each question.

Epidemiology/aetiology (Answers, p. 88)

1 The average general practice with 2000 patients will have about 50 diabetics.
2 5% of diagnosed diabetics are insulin dependent.
3 Indo-Asians have an incidence of diabetes double that of Caucasians.
4 30% of patients with impaired glucose tolerance will develop diabetes within 10 years.
5 In classical NIDDM beta-cells are slowly destroyed by an auto-immune process.

Discussion point

Does your practice or clinic have a diabetic register? Think of ways this might be established and kept up to date and how it might prove useful. Imagine that you are the Director of a city's diabetic service and your health authority has allocated you a further £100 000. How might a diabetic register help you spend the money appropriately? See Skill Topic 24 on Audit for ideas.

Diagnosis (Answers, p. 88)

1 Diabetes is diagnosed by the finding of 2% glycosuria.
2 A random venous plasma glucose of 11.1 mmol/l confirms the diagnosis of diabetes in a symptomatic patient.
3 A fasting venous plasma glucose of 6.8 mmol/l confirms the diagnosis of diabetes in a symptomatic patient.
4 Testing for glycosuria is an acceptable screening test for diabetes in the general population.

Clinical scenario

Question. A 47 year old asymptomatic Caucasian female attends a private health screen. You are notified that her random blood glucose is 9.3 mmol/l. What would you do and how quickly would you do it?
Answer: This level of blood glucose is not diagnostic of diabetes. A glucose tolerance test is required. Presuming that the patient is asymptomatic a delay of up to 10 days would be acceptable.

Initial management (Answers, p. 89)

1 Newly diagnosed diabetics with ketonuria should be admitted to hospital.

2 The decision to start insulin is determined by the severity of hyperglycaemia.

3 NIDDM patients can be given a trial of diet alone even if symptomatic.

4 In asymptomatic NIDDM patients the initial trial of diet should last 12 weeks.

5 A fasting venous plasma glucose of 8 mmol/l would necessitate starting an OHA after a 12 week trial diet.

6 Patients under the age of 30 always require insulin from diagnosis.

Practice point

In the midst of a busy surgery a patient who has attended because of tiredness mentions a dry mouth. Your feeling of self-congratulation for remembering to test the urine passes rapidly into one of terror as the urine testing strip changes colour from blue to green to brown. Don't panic. First establish the diagnosis (Skill Sheet 1) and then take it step by step by following the flow chart (Skill Sheets 2 and 3). It is unwise to delay, do a finger prick blood glucose test on the spot with a venous plasma blood glucose and U & Es phoned back the same day from the lab.

Diet (Answers, p. 89)

1 In the diabetic diet carbohydrates should supply at least 50% of energy requirements.

2 Slowly absorbed foods such as beans and lentils should be avoided as they make diabetic control difficult.

3 Rapidly absorbed sugar foods, e.g. sweets, chocolate or sweet drinks, should never be taken except during a 'hypo'.

4 The intake of sugar should be kept as near to zero as possible.

5 Low calorie squashes, diet fizzy drinks and artificial sweeteners are recommended for diabetics.

6 Special 'diabetic foods' containing sorbitol and fructose are a useful adjunct to the diabetic diet.

7 Insulin treated patients require snacks between meals and at bedtime to prevent hypoglycaemia.

8 The carbohydrate exchange system is mandatory for all insulin dependent diabetics.

9 Patients on insulin can be advised that it is acceptable to take up to 21 units (male) or 14 units (female) of alcohol per week.

10 A sensible weight loss target for the obese NIDDM patient is 1–2 kg/month.

11 The recommended intake of fibre for diabetics is 30 g/day.

Practice point

Leaflets produced by the British, Australian or American Diabetes Associations contain valuable and comprehensive guidance which in most cases is no more than you will need to know for day to day management. It is worth viewing these so that you and your patients are working from similar information bases. It is recommended that all patients with diabetes should be seen by a dietician.

Oral hypoglycaemic agents (Answers, p. 90)

1 Metformin is a sulphonylurea.
2 Chlorpropramide is particularly liable to cause hypoglycaemia.
3 Metformin causes hypoglycaemia at high therapeutic doses.
4 Tolbutamide is always given once daily.
5 Metformin is suitable for obese patients.
6 Metformin should not be prescribed for normal weight patients even if in combination with a sulphonylurea.
7 Metformin can be used safely in alcoholics.
8 After a 12 week dietary trial the majority of newly diagnosed NIDDM patients will require the addition of an OHA.
9 Sulphonylureas aid weight loss.
10 Acarbose delays absorption of glucose.

Remember

Always check renal function before starting an OHA. In renal impairment metformin can cause lactic acidosis and renally excreted sulphonylureas may cause hypoglycaemia. However, tolbutamide and gliclazide are principally metabolised by the liver and can be used in renal impairment.

Insulin (Answers, p. 91)

1 Soluble insulin (clear) has a duration of action of 12–24 hours.
2 Absorption of insulin is affected by the site at which it is administered.
3 Soluble insulin can be mixed with isophane insulin.
4 The basal bolus regimen is suitable for the elderly as it involves just one injection per day.

5 Patients on twice daily injections of a premixed insulin of soluble and isophane should adjust their insulin dosage from day to day according to their SBGM.
6 Routine insulin dosage adjustments for poor control should be of the order of 10% up or down.
7 An isolated severe hypoglycaemic reaction should prompt an immediate reduction in insulin.
8 A high fasting blood sugar for several days in a patient on a twice daily premixed insulin requires an increase in the morning insulin.
9 When drawing up insulin, always draw up the clear (soluble) insulin first.
10 When injecting insulin the skin should be 'pinched up'.
11 When injecting insulin the needle should be inserted at right-angles to the skin.
12 Maximum insulin sensitivity occurs in the evening.
13 Research has now conclusively proved an association between hypoglycaemia and switching to human insulin.
14 Insulin pens have not been shown to improve overall diabetic control.
15 Patients usually require approximately three-fifths of total dose of insulin in the morning.

Practice point

The most important point about adjusting insulin is that a persistently inadequate blood glucose at a particular time of day requires adjustment of the prior insulin dose. Therefore, if high early in the morning then alter the evening long-acting insulin, if high before lunch adjust morning short-acting insulin, if high at teatime adjust morning long-acting insulin, and if high last thing at night adjust evening short-acting insulin.

Monitoring (Answers, p. 92)

1 Fasting blood sugar is a good measure of overall control in IDDM.
2 The amount of HbA1 in the circulation corresponds to mean glycaemia over the 60 days half life of the red blood cell.
3 Blood loss and haemolysis can give a spuriously high HbA1.
4 Patients should consult their doctor or diabetic nurse specialist if their blood glucose is >20 mmol/l for 4 days or more.
5 With SBGM it is best to test 2 hours after a meal.

NIDDM and insulin (Answers, p. 93)

1 NIDDM patients on maximal oral therapy who have moderate hyperglycaemia with symptoms such as lethargy and general weakness are
likely to be helped by insulin therapy.
2 When switching an NIDDM patient to insulin it is best to start with
soluble insulin alone as the effects are not prolonged and dosage adjustments are easily made.
3 Most cases of OHA failure are in fact due to poor dietary compliance.
4 A regimen combining insulin and metformin can be used in obese
NIDDM patients.

Retinopathy (Answers, p. 93)

1 Retinal haemorrhages are a feature of background retinopathy.
2 If the visual acuities are normal there is unlikely to be any serious diabetes induced pathology within the eye requiring eye clinic
referral.
3 The macula is situated 2 disc widths medial to the disc.
4 Maculopathy is the commonest cause of visual impairment in patients
with diabetes.
5 Visual loss due to maculopathy only occurs when there are exudates on
the macula.
6 If pain occurs some hours following the use of 1% Tropicamide it is
likely to be due to an irritant reaction and an alternative mydriatic
should be found.

7 The new vessels of proliferative retinopathy can cause both vitreous and retinal detachments.
8 Once serious retinopathy is established better diabetic control cannot prevent its progress.

> **Back to basics**
> Retinal screening is a skilled task requiring training and practice. Start with the most basic task: testing visual acuity. See Appendix 2 and check whether the procedures outlined are followed correctly in your practice or clinic.

Diabetic nephropathy (Answers, p. 94)
1 Diabetic nephropathy develops in up to 20–30% of IDDM patients after 20 years.
2 Serum creatinine is a good marker of the early stages of impaired renal function in diabetic nephropathy.
3 The finding of proteinuria (Albustix positive) in the absence of other causes such as a urinary infection suggests diabetic nephropathy.
4 Patients with diabetic nephropathy should be referred for specialist care if their creatinine rises above normal.
5 Tight glycaemic control affects progression of established nephropathy.
6 Haematuria is usual in diabetic nephropathy.

> **Clinical scenario**
> A 25 year old insulin dependant diabetic is found to have a trace of proteinuria at routine check-up.
> What action should you take?
> See Skill Topics 10, Microalbuminuria & 11, Diabetic nephropathy for guidance.

Diabetic neuropathy (Answers, p. 94)
1 Can occur acutely.
2 Can be painful.
3 Is always bilateral.
4 Can cause an 'irritable' or neurogenic bladder.
5 Can cause vomiting.
6 Troublesome neuropathy can be reversed by good glycaemic control.
7 The prevalence of impotence in male patients may be as high as 40%.
8 Testing for light touch with cotton wool is the best way to detect diabetic neuropathy.

Foot problems (Answers, p. 94)

1 Diabetic foot problems are an important cause of diabetic in-patient care.
2 Diabetic foot ulcers are preventable.
3 The typical 'diabetic foot' is usually cold unless infected.
4 The typical 'diabetic foot' is excessively moist and sweaty.
5 A diabetic whose foot becomes warm and swollen after episodes of minor trauma is likely to have an early Charcot joint.
6 Diabetes with ulcers penetrating to deep tissue layers should be referred to hospital even if apyrexial.
7 Doppler studies of peripheral blood flow are unlikely to be helpful in the management of diabetic foot problems.

Hypertension and diabetes (Answers, p. 95)

1 Reduction of blood pressure slows decline of renal function in patients with diabetic nephropathy.
2 ACE inhibitors have a protective effect on the kidneys of patients with diabetic nephropathy which is independent of their antihypertensive effect.
3 ACE inhibitors have no effect on the kidneys of normotensive patients with microalbuminuria.
4 Thiazide diuretics in low dose (1.25 or 2.5 mg) have minimal metabolic effects.
5 ACE inhibitors are less effective in Afro-Caribbeans.
6 Thiazide diuretics are less effective in renal impairment.
7 Beta blockers remain a good first line choice for IDDM hypertensives.

8 Alpha blockers can be used safely with other anti-hypertensive agents.
9 The major threat to hypertensive NIDDM patients is renal failure.
10 NIDDM with microalbuminuria or other evidence of end organ damage should be treated if their blood pressure is greater than 140/90.

Audit suggestion

A recent expert consensus statement advocates a more aggressive approach to blood pressure management. Our own latest general practice based audit demonstrated an unexpected number of patients with untreated blood pressure recordings above the treatment thresholds indicated in Skill Topic 15, Hypertension and diabetes. See how many of your diabetic patients have raised blood pressure and how many are on therapy. You may be surprised at the result.

Lipids and diabetes (Answers, p. 96)

1 Reduced HDL levels are a typical feature of NIDDM. See scenario 9.
2 The hypertriglyceridaemia often seen in diabetics (particularly NIDDM) is resistant to improvements made in glycaemic control.
3 The recommendations for the treatment of hyperlipidaemia in diabetics are based on the results of lipid lowering trials in diabetic populations.
4 For diabetic patients without IHD who have moderately raised cholesterol and triglycerides the treatment of choice is a fibrate or atorvastatin.
5 Diabetics with hypercholesterolaemia will need to alter their diabetic diet substantially to incorporate lipid lowering features.

Hypoglycaemia (Answers, p. 96)

1 In the correction of hypoglycaemia 50 ml of glucose based drink will provide 10 g of carbohydrate.
2 Following correction of hypoglycaemia with a rapid-acting carbohydrate, e.g. a glucose based drink, no further food should be given until the next scheduled snack or meal.

Practice point

In patients who are going through a phase of oscillating poor control with frequent severe 'hypos' and unpredictably high blood glucose results try, if necessary by insulin adjustment, to correct the hypos first. This is the patient's most pressing need. Once this is done efforts can be made to improve overall control.

---

3 Loss of warning signs of hypoglycaemia can persist for 1 week after a severe hypoglycaemia attack.
4 Hypoglycaemia is uncommon in patients on sulphonylureas.

Intercurrent illness (Answers, p. 96)

1 A patient on insulin who has a pyrexial illness should have the insulin dosage decreased by 10–20% to prevent hypoglycaemia.
2 During illness toast and honey is a suitable substitute for a normal meal.
3 Hospital admission is indicated if there are any ketones in the urine.
4 Patients on OHAs whose blood glucose is >20 mmol/l for more than 24 hours during an intercurrent illness should be considered for short term insulin therapy.

Practice point
It goes against the grain for diabetics to drink sugary 'pop' at any time, but when they are ill with a diminished solid food intake, this is what they may have to do to maintain even control. Look carefully at the practical guidelines in Skill Topic 17, Intercurrent illness.

Administrative matters (Answers, p. 97)

1 To fulfil the requirements of the Chronic Disease Management Programme for Diabetes a general practitioner must review his or her diabetic patients every 6 months.
2 Clinical audit is a compulsory feature of the diabetic Chronic Disease Management Programme.
3 The fee to a general practitioner for organising the diabetic Chronic Disease Management programme is calculated on the basis of the number of hours likely to be devoted to it.
4 General practitioners are required to keep a register of diabetic patients whether or not they are receiving the Chronic Disease Management fee.
5 Single-handed general practitioners may carry out a diabetic Chronic Disease Management Programme jointly with other general practitioners to pool resources and still each be paid a full fee.

Epidemiology/aetiology

1 TRUE. Increasing incidence makes this often quoted figure a conservative estimate. A proportion (approximately 15) of these patients will be undiagnosed. Incidence increases as population ages.

2 FALSE. 15%. The incidence of IDDM is doubling every 20 years in the UK.

3 FALSE. 4–5 times higher. The proportion of Indo-Asians in the English Midlands city of Leicester with diabetes is 11% for those age 45–65 and up to 20% for those age over 65.

4 TRUE. So it's worth doing a yearly postprandial blood glucose on patients with impaired glucose tolerance. Remember that impaired glucose tolerance is diagnosed by a glucose tolerance test.

5 FALSE. In classical NIDDM there is initially hyperinsulinism, often precipitated by obesity and insulin resistance. Eventually the pancreas becomes 'worn out' and insulin production falls. A proportion (approximately 15%) of NIDDM patients have a variable degree of autoimmune destruction.

NIDDM, along with obesity, hyperlipidaemia and hypertension, forms one part of the so-called syndrome 'X' or insulin resistance syndrome, a cluster of risk factors strongly associated with coronary heart disease.

Diagnosis

1 FALSE. Confirmation by blood tests is required. Renal glycosuria is not uncommon and erroneous diagnosis has enormous social and financial implications.

2 TRUE. No need to proceed to a glucose tolerance test. Asymptomatic patients require two abnormal random values.

3 FALSE. A value of >7.0 mmol/l is diagnostic. It is worth reviewing the diagnostic criteria on Skill Topic 1. It is surprising how often misdiagnosis or inappropriate glucose tolerance tests are performed.

4 TRUE. A good way to screen larger numbers, e.g. at a well-person clinic. A 3 yearly postprandial venous plasma glucose has been suggested for those with a positive family history, Indo-Asians, previous gestational diabetes or previous hyperglycaemia in illness. Remember

that diabetes is a great diagnostic deceiver and that there will be few practitioners who have not 'missed' a case by failing to test the urine. Think of diabetes in patients with:

cataracts;

enuresis;

recurrent infections;

impotence;

weight loss;

angina/peripheral vascular disease;

pruritus;

tiredness;

thrush;

hypertension.

Initial management

1 FALSE. The criteria for hospital admissions are clinical: dehydration, vomiting, pyrexia, disordered breathing, hypotension, drowsiness, etc.

2 FALSE. Insulin deficiency is implied by moderate or severe ketonuria or by weight loss, not by a particular level of blood glucose. Conversely, a patient with only moderate hyperglycaemia but moderate to severe ketosis will require insulin.

3 TRUE. See Skill Topic 3, Initial management flow chart. There is disagreement over *how long* a symptomatic patient should be expected to diet, before therapy is started. A 12 week trial is ideal but if the patient is non-obese *or* fasting glucose remains above 15 mmol/l *or* marked symptoms persist drug therapy may be started earlier. Try and review patients frequently in the early weeks after diagnosis.

4 TRUE. Then assess control with a fasting venous plasma glucose and/or HbA1. Inadequate trial of diet is a common fault in diabetic management leading to the unnecessary early introduction of oral hypoglycaemic agents.

5 TRUE. 7 mmol/l is an acceptable cut off (or HbA1 greater than normal range). A higher level is acceptable in the elderly. See Skill Topic 8, Targets for control.

6 FALSE. A small proportion of patients have maturity onset diabetes of young (MODY). They do not have weight loss or ketonuria and require insulin only if metabolic control is poor.

Diet

1 TRUE. This is considerably higher than in the average person's diet in the UK, although such a diet can equally be advised for the non-diabetic. For a person taking a 2500 calorie diet this recommendation

translates into a large amount of carbohydrate; 8 slices of bread, 4 potatoes, 1 portion of macaroni, 2 cups of breakfast cereal or porridge, as well as portions of milk, fruit, peas and beans would be required to make up the daily quantity. In practice it means a drastic reduction in fats and oils and much smaller portions of meat, fish and cheese than we are all used to eating.

2 FALSE. These foods have a low 'glycaemic index' and therefore avoid the high peaks of glucose release.

3 FALSE. They can be taken before vigorous exercise and some flexibility is advised for special occasions particularly with children. Remember, glucose itself is not harmful, only when it is high in the blood.

4 FALSE. Up to 25 g of added sugar per day is permitted providing that the patient is (a) not obese (b) it is spread through the day and (c) it is taken in conjunction with high fibre, high starch foods. Ever tried baking using no sugar at all?

5 TRUE. Aspartame is particularly suitable. Sorbitol, as used in 'diabetic foods' tends to cause diarrhoea.

6 FALSE. May be glucose free but are just as calorific and very expensive.

7 TRUE. Particularly if they are on soluble insulin. An apple, muesli bar, a round of wholemeal toast, a packet of low fat crisps (30 g) are examples of appropriate snacks.

8 FALSE. It can be used, but nowadays it is considered more important that each meal provides a balance of complex carbohydrates with limited amounts of protein and fat. How good are you at remembering what you have eaten and how good is your counting?

9 TRUE. The important exceptions here are that obese diabetics are unlikely to lose weight if they drink this amount, that alcohol can exacerbate hypoglycaemia and that liqueurs and sweet wines should be avoided. It is sensible to reduce this limit to 9 units per week in patients with poor control. Do you know how many calories a glass of wine contains?

10 TRUE. More attainable than the depressing 'you need to lose 15 kg'.

11 TRUE. But this is twice that currently taken in the UK diet. 30 g of fibre amounts to just over 7 portions of foods such as a round of wholemeal bread, peas, beans, wholemeal pasta, sprouts, bran flakes, muesli, etc. A daunting task!

Oral hypoglycaemic agents

1 FALSE. It is a biguanide. If you get this wrong you need an urgent read of the relevant section of your local formulary or pharmacological textbook.

2 TRUE. This drug is principally excreted by the kidney and since renal function declines with age, there is a tendency for it to accumulate. Thus, this drug is rarely used now due to its long duration of action.

3 FALSE. Other side-effects yes, such as nausea or diarrhoea but *not* hypoglycaemia. One of its advantages.

4 FALSE. Can be given once daily initially but is more frequently administered thrice daily before meals. Particularly suitable for the elderly if compliance can be assured because of its short half-life (excreted principally by the liver).

5 TRUE. Its main indication. Can be used in combination with insulin.

6 FALSE. Combination therapy is useful if sulphonylureas in maximum dosage are not achieving satisfactory control. See Scenario 7.

7 FALSE. Due to increased susceptibility to lactic acidosis. Avoid also in cardiac and renal failure.

8 TRUE. Only a minority will achieve a fasting plasma glucose of <7 mmol/l.

9 FALSE. Unfortunately sulphonylureas encourage weight gain. An adequate trial of diet is preferable before starting them.

10 FALSE. It inhibits the enzymatic digestion of sucrose and starch. Hence glucose and not sucrose should be used if hypoglycaemia occurs when acarbose is used in combination with a sulphonylurea.

Insulin

1 FALSE. Peak activity 2–5 hours, onset after $\frac{1}{2}$ hour.

2 TRUE. Insulin is absorbed more rapidly from the arm than from the abdomen than from the buttock than from the thigh.

3 TRUE. But not with zinc suspensions.

4 FALSE. One injection at night of a long- or intermediate-acting insulin with soluble insulin thrice daily at meal times. See Skill Topic 7, Insulin therapy. Remember, it does not always lead to better control and can allow the occasional patient to manipulate the dose four times a day!

5 FALSE. This will result in unstable, oscillating control. Assess the profiles taken over several days and then adjust the dose.

6 TRUE. 2–4 units is usually appropriate.

7 FALSE. There is usually an explanation such as a missed snack, unaccustomed exercise or change of injection site. Remember, only adjust insulin dose on the basis of trends.

8 FALSE. An increase in evening insulin is required (unless you suspect the patient may be having nocturnal hypoglycaemia, in which case the evening dose should be *reduced*).

9 TRUE. In order not to contaminate the soluble insulin bottle with the longer acting insulins. Sequence is:

1 Inject air into cloudy bottle.

2 Inject air into clear bottle.

3 Draw up clear.

4 Draw up cloudy.

10 TRUE. Otherwise could have an i.m. injection which is painful. Insulin is always injected subcutaneously.

11 TRUE. Less painful and prevents an intradermal injection. The only exception is in young thin patients who are injecting into the arm when the injection may have to be at 45 degrees to avoid going into muscle.

12 FALSE. Around 3 a.m. For this reason too much isophane insulin at tea or bedtime may cause a 3 a.m. 'hypo', followed by reactive pre-breakfast hyperglycaemia, the so-called Somogyi effect. For patients on fixed ratio insulin combinations this problem can be difficult to address without upsetting control at a different time. Sometimes it is necessary to switch patients to a regimen using separate short- and intermediate-acting insulins so that adjustments are more 'tailor-made'. This sort of change needs to be made by a diabetologist.

13 FALSE. Human insulins are less immunogenic with a more rapid action and shorter duration of action but have not been shown to cause more hypoglycaemia. However, the BDA states that patients who report problems should not be discouraged from switching back to animal insulin if problems occur and they request it.

14 TRUE. Very convenient and well accepted but still the same insulin! The pen's short, fine 30G neeedle can be a useful advantage especially in children.

15 TRUE.

Monitoring

1 FALSE. Too much day to day variation. It *is* a good measure in NIDDM patients on diet or OHAs.

2 TRUE. This is of obvious relevance when it comes to deciding how often to measure HbA1. More often than every 3 months is unnecessary.

3 FALSE. Spuriously low. Think about it. Red cell half life is reduced so there will be less HbA1. HbA1 spuriously high in uraemia.

4 TRUE. They should consult earlier and at a lower level of blood glucose (>15 mmol/l) if they feel ill, are vomiting or have a fever. The general practitioner should remember to test for ketones.

5 FALSE. The majority of tests should be fasting or preprandial with a lesser number done postprandial or at bed time.

NIDDM and insulin

1 TRUE. An indication for starting insulin. Up to 70% of patients report a beneficial effect on well-being after transfer to insulin.

2 FALSE. Isophane (intermediate action) insulin is required. Relatively easy to adjust and suitable for NIDDM. Because many patients require the addition of a soluble component some diabetologists start insulin therapy using a premixed insulin.

3 FALSE. The natural history of NIDDM is for the beta cells to eventually 'wear out'. If this happens then it is pointless to insist on weight loss. To make matters complicated there are some patients for whom successful dieting can reduce insulin resistance and thus improve control. Deciding whether or not a patient's diet is adequate is difficult and in practice a formal review of diet by a dietician is often helpful before starting insulin.

4 TRUE. This can be a difficult group of patients as insulin can stimulate appetite and increase obesity thus causing a vicious circle of increased insulin needs and poor control. Metformin or, alternatively, acarbose may help prevent weight gain and review by a dietician will also help.

Retinopathy

1 TRUE. Typically 'dot' or 'blot'.

2 FALSE. There may be perimacular exudates with encroaching oedema threatening imminent and preventable damage to the macula. Proliferative retinopathy can be present at an advanced stage without deterioration of the eyesight until a vitreous haemorrhage occurs.

3 FALSE. Lateral or temporal.

4 TRUE. Particularly in NIDDM patients. The visual impairment of maculopathy does not improve using a pin hole (in contrast to a refractive error).

5 FALSE. Circinate exudates (exudates within 1 disc diameter of the centre of the macula often in a ring like formation) can cause visual loss due to macular oedema.

6 FALSE. Could be due to acute glaucoma. Tropicamide can cause slight stinging for up to 60 sec following insertion.

7 TRUE. Two of the ways proliferative retinopathy impair sight. The others are by fibrous tissue and by haemorrhage.

8 TRUE. But good glycaemic control is preventative and will slow the rate of progression of existing retinopathy in the earlier stages. The three main factors in the development of retinopathy are hypertension, degree of hyperglycaemia and duration of diabetes.

Diabetic nephropathy

1 TRUE. The incidence has been declining in recent decades.
2 FALSE. It only rises when the GFR has fallen to 50% of normal.
3 TRUE. Absence of retinopathy is often quoted as a clue that proteinuria may be due to other pathology and that renal biopsy is indicated.
4 TRUE. By this time glomerular filtration rate has fallen significantly.
5 FALSE. Unfortunately not. However, aggressive blood pressure control does affect the progression of established nephropathy. (See Skill Topic 15, Hypertension and diabetes.)
6 FALSE. Other pathology should be sought (although microscopic haematuria can occur).

Diabetic neuropathy

1 TRUE. Sometimes at diagnosis or after a period of hyperglycaemia or during intercurrent illness. Occasionally precipitated just after insulin is started.
2 TRUE. Definitely yes. Often causes marked debility and needs treatment with low dose tricyclics or carbamezapine as well as analgesics. Often difficult to treat.
3 FALSE. The mononeuropathies such as diabetic amyotrophy are usually unilateral.
4 FALSE. Atonic bladder, enlarged, with overflow.
5 TRUE. Autonomic neuropathy can cause gastric paresis.
6 FALSE. Prevented, yes. Reversed, unfortunately no. The exception to this is the acute painful neuropathy associated with hyperglycaemia.
7 TRUE. Important to ask, although it may not be appropriate to have a tick box on your shared care card. There have been considerable recent advances so consider specialist referral.
8 FALSE. Light touch can be preserved until a late stage and indeed hypersensitivity can be a problem early on. It is wise to test also for pin-prick and vibration sense with a 128c tuning fork.

Foot problems

1 TRUE. Once established they are slow to heal and so often require long periods of admission. However, the use of specialist footwear, such as the Scotchcast boot, which protect the ulcer from pressure and allow the patient to remain ambulatory reduce the number of days in hospital.
2 TRUE. Education and screening programmes have been shown to reduce the risk of ulcers developing.
3 FALSE. Autonomic neuropathy leads to increased skin blood flow unless there is gross large vessel disease.

4 FALSE. Due to autonomic neuropathy, it is more likely to be dry, leading to thin, easily cracked skin.

5 TRUE. X-ray or bone scans are useful investigations to pick up destructive or hypertrophic changes.

6 TRUE. Debridement and non-weight bearing techniques are likely to be necessary.

7 FALSE. Diabetic ulcers do not heal in the presence of ischaemia. Doppler studies have become an essential part of the assessment. Remember, you may be caught out thinking that the warm foot due to autonomic neuropathy has a good blood supply.

Hypertension and diabetes

1 TRUE. No matter which agent is used.

2 TRUE. ACE inhibitors have been shown to halve the combined risk of death, requirement for dialysis and transplantation in patients with nephropathy and hypertension.

3 FALSE. Still under investigation but there is increasing evidence that ACE inhibitors prevent or postpone the development of diabetic nephropathy in normotensive patients with microalbuminuria.

4 TRUE. Few glycaemic or dyslipidaemic effects but may cause or exacerbate impotence.

5 TRUE. A calcium antagonist or an alpha blocker is the drug of choice.

6 TRUE. Loop diuretics are more often used in this situation if a diuretic is required at all.

7 FALSE. Three good reasons why not:
  1 May mask hypoglycaemia.
  2 Mild adverse effects on lipid profile.
  3 Exacerbation of limb ischaemia problems.
  But they may still be used if ischaemic heart disease is a problem.

8 TRUE. But they should be introduced slowly to avoid postural hypotension. They have the advantage of being lipid neutral and metabolic neutral.

9 FALSE. Cardiovascular disease is still the biggest problem. Most NIDDM patients succumb to the ravages of vascular diseases before renal failure has time to develop.

10 TRUE. Caution is required in the elderly and those with macrovascular disease particularly if using ACE inhibitors. Atherosclerotic renal artery stenosis may predispose the patient to rapid deterioration in renal function so it is important to always check renal function before and 7–14 days after starting an ACE inhibitor.

Lipids and diabetes

1 TRUE. One of the cluster of risk factors for coronary heart disease which includes also insulin resistance, hyperglycaemia, hypertension and hypertriglyceridaemia.

2 FALSE. Important catch. Improve diabetic control before rushing in with lipid lowering agents. The treatment of isolated hypertriglyceridaemia is controversial (>4.5 mmol/l).

3 FALSE. The recommendations are based on evidence predominantly from trials in non-diabetic patients and extrapolate their findings on the basis of the high cardiovascular risk evident in diabetics. The situation should be clearer once the United Kingdom Propective Diabetes Study (UKPDS) and the Collaborative Atorvastatin Diabetes Study (CARDS) have been published.

4 TRUE. Most experts recommend that diabetics should be prescribed the same drugs as non-diabetics.

5 FALSE. The diabetic diet and lipid lowering diet are very similar and patients become very confused if they feel they are on 'two diets'. Reinforcement of advice already given is more appropriate, emphasising the low fat elements.

Hypoglycaemia

1 TRUE. Most 'hypos' require approximately 20 g of carbohydrate. It is important to have a rough idea of how much is needed to correct a 'hypo'. See Skill Topic 18, Hypoglycaemia.

2 FALSE. It is important to follow up with some slow-release carbohydrate, e.g. an apple, or toast, or a bowl of cereal. Long-acting insulin could still be working and a second 'hypo' is possible. Remember also that vigorous exercise can cause increased insulin sensitivity for up to 12 hours after the exercise is finished.

3 TRUE. The loss is associated with tight glycaemic control and (in the absence of autonomic neuropathy) can be reversed by a period of less strict control. Also, loss of warning occurs in 30% of IDDM patients after 20 years of therapy.

4 FALSE. Surprisingly common, particularly for patients on chlorpropramide or glibenclamide with the risk of hypoglycaemia lasting for 24–48 hours. Admission to hospital is required for severe cases.

Intercurrent illness

1 FALSE. An increase in insulin requirements is much more likely to be needed due to a temporary rise in insulin resistance.

2 TRUE. Smaller quantities taken more frequently will be required.

3 FALSE. Moderate or severe ketonuria demands hospital admission,

smaller amounts permit home management with frequent review providing the clinical condition of the patient is satisfactory. Remember, the clinical condition of the patient is often the most important factor in deciding whether hospital admission is necessary.

4 TRUE. They will feel better, and get better quicker. Hospital admission would be required.

Administrative matters

1 FALSE. At least annually. Requirements are for 'a full review of the patient's health including checks for potential complications and a review of the patient's own monitoring needs'.

2 TRUE. See Red Book para 30, schedule 4, item 10 (Audit).

3 FALSE At a current fee per general practitioner of £395 this could not be so. The fee is designed as an incentive to provide the programme.

4 TRUE. A little known amendment (1993) to the terms of service stated that a general practitioner must include in his annual report the number of patients on his list who are diabetic.

5 TRUE. Some complicated Red Book hocus pocus here.

For full details see para 30, schedule 4 of The Red Book.

If you are not a British general practitioner you can ignore this section.

The Diabetes Control and Complications Trial

The DCCT (*N Engl J Med* (1993) **329**, 977–86) is a landmark trial which concluded that 'Intensive insulin therapy effectively delays the onset and slows the progression of diabetic retinopathy, nephropathy and neuropathy in patients with IDDM'.

• 1441 IDDM patients were split into two groups, conventional management and intensive management (home blood glucose monitoring, education sessions, multiple injection regimen or pump).

• In patients free of retinopathy at entry the chances of developing it over the 6.5 years of the trial were 6% if intensively treated and 24% if conventionally treated.

• In patients with mild to moderate retinopathy the chances of it progressing were 21% if intensively treated and 47% if conventionally treated.

• Similarly impressive results were seen for neuropathy and only slightly less impressive results were seen for nephropathy.

• The important outcome was seen across the age group studied (ages 13–39).

• This was despite the fact that although mean HbA1C fell from 9% to 7% in the intensively treated group (equivalent to a fall from 11% to 9% using HbA1) only a minority reached the target HbA1C of 6% (HbA1 of 8%).

But

• There was a 3-fold increase in **severe** hypoglycaemia 'in which assistance was required in providing treatment' in the intensively treated group.

• Trial design excluded patients with previous severe hypoglycaemia or loss of warning symptoms. The incidence of hypoglycaemia is therefore likely to be underestimated.

• Intensively treated patients gained an average of 4.5 kg in weight more than the conventionally treated.

• Trial patients are likely to have been highly motivated; in ordinary practice, targets must be individualised, realistic and negotiated. Any improvement in control is likely to be helpful.

• Intensive treatment is inappropriate in children, the elderly and

those with widespread and advanced complications or hypoglycaemic unawareness.
- Most experts are willing to extrapolate the results to NIDDM patients.

The St Vincent's Declaration
In 1989, at St Vincent in Italy, a meeting of diabetes professionals and diabetes organisations set out a number of goals and targets for diabetic care. You may see the Declaration referred to and full details are available if you join the Professional Division of the BDA.
It is hoped to:
- Reduce new cases of blindness by one-third.
- Reduce end stage diabetic renal failure by one-third.
- Reduce limb amputation by one-half.
- Normalise outcome of pregnancy to non-diabetic level.
- Cut coronary heart disease morbidity and mortality.

How to test visual acuity

Equipment

A 6 metre Snellen chart with the patient 6 metres away. The chart must be well lit. If there is not enough space, use a reversed 6 metre chart with a mirror. The distance from the chart to the mirror and back to the patient should still be 6 metres. If you cannot do either of the above, use a 3 metre chart with the patient 3 metres away.

Method

1 Always explain to patients what you are doing. Do not hurry them.
2 Face them towards the chart at the correct distance.
3 Always test and record the right eye first to avoid confusion later.
4 If glasses or lenses are worn for distance then test wearing them.
   The aim is to record the best possible corrected vision.
5 Express the visual acuity as a fraction, e.g. $\frac{6}{12}$.
   The top figure represents the distance between the patient and the chart.
   The bottom figure represents the last complete line the patient can read.
   Normal vision is $\frac{6}{6}$, indicating the ability to read the 6 metre line from a distance of 6 metres.
6 If the visual acuity is $\frac{6}{9}$ or less, use the pin hole.
   Record visual acuity both without and with the pin hole.
   If glasses have been forgotten, use the pin hole.
7 Always record how the reading was obtained, i.e. unaided/ with glasses/ with pin hole.
8 If a patient is unable to read the top letter of the chart move them to 3 metres (record as $\frac{3}{n}$).
   If still unable to read the chart, proceed to counting fingers at 1 m (record as CF), or hand movements (record as HM).

   Any deterioration in visual acuity since the last test must be referred to the doctor.

   Reproduced by kind permission of David Taylor and Jane Perkins of the Exeter Diabetes and Vascular Health Centre and the British Diabetic Association, 10 Queen Anne Street, London W1M OBD. Tel: 0171 323 1531

Referral checklist

Who/what	Where	How soon
At diagnosis:		
• Patient ill with vomiting, dehydration, drowsiness or disordered breathing	Hospital admission	Immediate
• Patient needs Insulin or general practitioner unsure (see Skill Topic 2)	Consultant diabetologist	Same day discuss by phone
• NIDDM patient deteriorates in initial treatment phase, e.g. weight loss or ketonuria (see Skill Topic 2)	Consultant diabetologist	Same day discuss by phone
• Children (see Skill Topic 22)	Consultant paediatrician	Same day
• All patients	Dietician	Routine
Pregnant women (see Skill Topic 21)	Combined clinic	At 5 weeks' gestation by phone
Women wishing to conceive	Combined clinic	Routine
Adolescents	Diabetic clinic	Continual
Intercurrent illness		
• For advice on insulin dosage or food intake	Diabetic Specialist Nurse	Same day
• If patient ill with clinical concerns (see Skill Topic 17)	Hospital admission to diabetic team	Same day
Hypoglycaemia		
• If any factor likely to lead to prolonged 'hypo' (see Skill Topic 18)	Hospital admission	Immediate
Diabetic ketoacidosis Ketonuria ++ with hyperglycaemia	Hospital admission	Immediate

continued on p. 102

Continued

Who/what	Where	How soon
Feet:		
• Cellulitis or deep infection	Hospital admission	Same day
• New ulcers	Diabetic clinic or multidisciplinary foot clinic	Urgent
• High risk foot (see Skill Topic 13)	Multidisciplinary foot clinic	Routine
Eyes (see Skill Topic 9):		
• Unexplained drop in visual acuity of two lines or more of Snellen chart	Retinal clinic	Routine
• Background retinopathy and visual acuity worse than $\frac{6}{12}$ not correctable by spectacles or pin hole	Retinal clinic	Routine
• Maculopathy, preproliferative or proliferative retinopathy	Retinal clinic	Urgent
• Vitreous or pre-retinal haemorrhage or any other sudden loss of vision	Eye casualty	Immediate
Renal involvement (see Skill Topics 10, 11):		
• Creatinine above normal range	Diabetic clinic	Routine
• Confirmed microalbuminuria (see Skill Topic 10) and difficulty in achieving good levels of glycaemic and B.P control	Diabetic clinic	Routine
Neuropathy (see Skill Topic 12):		
• Pain	Diabetic clinic	Routine
• Severe autonomic		
Impotence (see Skill Topic 19)	Diabetic clinic	Routine
Failure to achieve satisfactory metabolic control and after discussion with patient (see Skill Topic 8):		
• IDDM	Diabetic clinic	Routine (depends on clinical condition)
• NIDDM, if consideration of insulin therapy	Diabetic clinic	Routine
• Both	Dietician	Routine

Quick learning planner

You are short of time . . . you need to cover the essentials fairly quickly. Here are 20 questions you can ask yourself cross-referenced to different parts of the teaching package. You may also find these useful if you have to cover the subject with a student or trainee.

1 What are the diagnostic criteria for diabetes mellitus?
    See Skill Topic 1

2 You test the urine of a child/adolescent/young adult/elderly person and it is 5% positive for sugar. What do you do next?
    See Questionnaire, Initial management, Skill Topics 2 & 3, Scenarios 1, 2 and 3.

3 What are the basics of the diabetic diet?
    See Questionnaire, Diet, Skill Topic 4, locally or nationally produced leaflets.

4 What are the main OHAs and when should they be used?
    See Questionnaire, Oral hypoglycaemic agents, Skill Topics 5 & 6.

5 How should patients adjust their insulin?
    See Questionnaire, Insulin, Scenarios 1 & 5.

6 How is hypoglycaemia treated?
    See Questionnaire, Hypoglycaemia, Skill Topic 18, Scenario 6.

7 What are the targets for biochemical control and what factors must be allowed for in their interpretation?
    See Questionnaire, Monitoring, Skill Topic 8, Scenario 7.

8 When and how should NIDDM patients be transferred onto insulin?
    See Skill Topic 7, Scenarios 4, 7 & 8.

9 How does the management of hypertension differ in diabetic patients?
    See Questionnaire, Hypertension, Skill Topic 15.

10 How do you examine the eye for diabetic complications and what are you looking for?
    See Questionnaire, Retinopathy, Skill Topic 6.

11 How do you examine the foot in diabetes and what are you looking for?
    See Questionnaire, Foot problems, Skill Topic 13, Scenario 10. Consult local or national patient leaflets.

12 In what way might diabetic neuropathy present clinically?
See Skill Topic 12, Scenario 10.
13 What is the natural history and clinical management of diabetic nephropathy?
See Questionnaire, Diabetic nephropathy, Skill Topic 11.
14 What is microalbuminuria, its significance and management?
See Skill Topic 10.
15 How is intercurrent illness managed in general practice?
See Questionnaire, Intercurrent illness, Skill Topic 17, Scenario 11.
16 How is the Chronic Disease Management Programme reimbursed?
See Para 30 of the Red Book.
17 How would you set up and run a general practice diabetic clinic?
See Scenarios 3 & 13.
18 What were the main findings of the DCCT?
See Appendix 1.
19 Why is close monitoring of diabetes essential in pregnancy?
See Skill Topic 21, Scenario 12.
20 What ideas would you have for a general practice diabetic audit and in what way could it be valuable?
See Skill Topic 24.

Useful addresses

British Diabetic Association
10 Queen Anne Street
London W1M 0BD
0171-323-1531

For a useful source of evidence based reviews:

Cochrane Library
Update Software
Summertown Pavilion
Middle Way
Summertown
Oxford OX2 7LG
01865 513902

International Diabetes Federation
1 rue Defacqz, 1000 Brussels
Belgium
00 32 2 538 5511

For copies of 'Medical Aspects of Fitness to Drive':

The Medical Commission on Accident Prevention
35–43 Lincoln's Inn Fields
London WC2A 3PN

Address for patients to notify about driving:

Medical Adviser,
Driver's Medical Unit
DVLA Longview Road
Swansea SA99 1TU
(Doctor's enquiry number at DVLA: 01792 783686)

(For information on state funded allowances such as Incapacity Benefit and Disability Living Allowance contact the local Social Security office, listed in the phone book under 'Benefits Agency').

For guidelines and protocols:

Royal College of General Practitioners,
14 Princes Gate, Hyde Park
London SW7 1PU
0171-581-3232

Royal College of Nursing
20 Cavendish Square
London W1M 0AB
0171-409-3333

Index